This book is written jointly by the founder of the Neal's Yard Remedies shops, Romy Fraser, and two of her colleagues, Susan Curtis and Irene Kohler, all of whom have many years experience in working with natural remedies. Susan Curtis runs a busy natural health practice.

Neal's Yard Remedies has made a huge impact since the first shop opened in Covent Garden, London. It is one of the pioneers of natural health care and natural beauty products.

# Neal's Yard Natural Remedies

*Susan Curtis, Romy Fraser, Irene Kohler*

Neal's Yard Press
16 Stambourne Way
West Wickham
Kent BR4 9NF

This fully revised and updated edition published in 2006 by
Neal's Yard Press

First published in Great Britain by Arkana 1988
Revised and reprinted by Penguin Books 1997

ISBN(10) 1-905830-00-9
(ISBN-13: 978-1-905830-00-8)

Printed by Biddles

Grateful thanks for their valuable contributions are offered to Dragana Vilinac and Julie Wood.

# CONTENTS

# INTRODUCTION

We opened our first Neal's Yard Remedies shop in 1981, and very much feel that we have been part of the enormous change and growth of natural medicines and therapies since that time. Our policy was then and is still the same now: to inform our customers what the various remedies available are for and help you to choose what you feel best suits your symptoms.

Our policy of telling customers what the various remedies are for and helping them to choose for themselves does two things. Firstly, it helps people to find a remedy that will bring them relief, and secondly, it gives people the knowledge they need to feel more empowered to look after themselves. This has been a quiet revolution, the evidence of which is the growth of the company and the fact that it is now the norm to use an herbal, homœopathic or other natural remedy by the majority of the population in the UK.

Making our own decisions is the best way to learn, and using this book will help you to do this. It gives you options for a large number of ailments from the three main areas of natural medicine: herbs, homœopathy and essential oils. The book has stood the test of time as being sensible and reliable. This 2006 edition has been revised and updated, but the information is essentially the same and in the same format.

What we hope we have achieved in this book is to give some ideas of safe and helpful remedies for common illness and first-aid. Much of our ill health is a result of the way we live, combined with inherited factors. The book is in the form of a simple alphabetical repertory; but always, any chosen remedy should be cross-referenced by consulting the appropriate specialist books that we recommend in the Further Reading, to get a more complete picture of the remedy itself and its appropriateness for the complaint. This particular book is one step in a learning process, a quest for health.

1

The whole question of ill-health and well-being is interesting.

Why should we get ill? Whose responsibility is it? And what can we learn from it? Maybe if we had been more in touch with our bodies and noticed the odd warnings that we received, we would have avoided the greater discomfort that we often find ourselves in. We may enjoy a few drinks, occasional junk food, running a home, and/or a demanding job, yet we continue to expect ourselves to remain fit, stress-free, and happy.

Encouraging our bodies towards an improved balance in health may involve changing our lifestyles. Do we want to do this? How much is it worth perpetuating a lifestyle that disturbs our well-being? Pollution, fast foods with additives, and the stress accumulated by the current values of society are continually pulling against a state of good health.

The process of becoming healthy offers the opportunity for growth and change. At times this process can be hindered or blocked by illness. In this book we can only offer solutions to some acute problems that are often the outcome of a temporary imbalance. When attitudes become fixed, then chronic complaints become established, and for these we will always recommend professional advice.

Something common to us all is the desire or drive to improve our lives, so here in this book our intention is to offer you the opportunity to take greater responsibility for your own discomfort or ill-health in a way that is safe and effective, but without the side-effects encountered when using synthetic drugs.

# HERBS

Plants are an integral part of the cycle of life on this planet. Human beings entirely depend on plant life to sustain us: not only are plants the source of all our food, but they create the air we breathe and are the original source of all our medicines. As life has become more complicated so too have the medicines we use. Modern society has largely replaced the use of healing plants — herbs — by sophisticated drugs. Currently, vast financial resources are being invested in the exploration and analysis of medicinal substances, often derivatives and synthetics based on plant constituents. However, in recent times, there is also a trend towards re-evaluating 'natural' medicine, and herbs are again being sought out for their intrinsic therapeutic properties.

The use of herbal medicine has been passed down through the centuries by those practiced in the art of healing. These traditional remedies are coming to be sought after again as effective, safe and proven alternatives to our synthetic medicines; and clinical trials are backing up traditional knowledge. Herbs can be used to support the natural healing processes in the body; not just directly attacking the disease, which is the approach generally offered by modern drugs.

For minor ailments the herbs that we suggest may be tried, but for real benefit in more serious cases a qualified herbalist should be consulted, who can assess each case individually and adjust the prescription and dosage as required.

## GATHERING HERBS

Many of the herbs we have recommended in this book can be found growing wild. Be certain that you are collecting the right species; some plants that look similar to useful herbs may be poisonous (use a field guide such as "The Medicinal Flora of Britain and Northwest Europe" by Julian Barker). Care must be taken that they are collected some distance from roads and any other sources of pollution. Gather only enough for your immediate use and do not dig up the roots; it is illegal to dig up any wild plants in the UK due to conservation issues.

Herbs can of course also be cultivated if you are lucky enough to have a garden, and then collected and used when needed.

To dry herbs gather them just before they have fully developed, in dry weather, as soon as the dew has gone in the morning. Remove any dead or damaged parts of the plants and then spread the herbs out to dry in a dry, well-ventilated atmosphere.

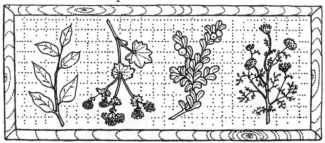

## STORAGE

Storage of your own herbs, or the ones that you purchase, should be away from light and in airtight jars. The effectiveness of herbalism depends greatly on the quality of the herbs used: they should look and smell fresh and bright.

## PREPARING HERBS

### INFUSIONS

An infusion is made like tea, it is the suitable method for herbal mixtures of flowers, leaves and green stems. Place the herb or herbs in a pot, pour on boiling water, cover and leave to stand for ten minutes before straining.

The quantity of herb to use will vary according to the quality of the herb and the strength of the infusion required. A general guide is to use one tablespoon of herbs to a pint of boiling water, or one heaped teaspoon of herbs to a cupful of boiling water. When using fresh herbs double the quantity of herb to be used.

Herbal preparations can be taken hot or cold. Hot infusions will tend to encourage sweating, cold ones tend to be more diuretic. Therefore, use hot infusions to treat colds, 'flu, fevers etc., these may be sweetened with honey for taste. If in doubt, it is usually considered best to take medicinal teas hot.

## DECOCTIONS

For the harder, woodier roots and barks of plants it is necessary to make a decoction. Place the herb or herbs in a saucepan, pour on some water, bring to the boil and then simmer for ten to fifteen minutes before straining. Do not use an aluminium pan but a glass, ceramic or unchipped enamel one. This method is also suitable for berries and the harder seeds.

Use the same quantities as recommended for infusions although you may need to add a little more water to allow for evaporation.

## TINCTURES

Alcohol-based preparations are called tinctures. Tinctures tend to be stronger, volume for volume, than infusions or decoctions. Dosage is normally between 1ml to 3ml of tincture taken in a wine glass of water. 1ml is roughly 25 drops.

## COMPRESSES AND POULTICES

To make a compress, use a clean cloth and soak it in a hot infusion or decoction. Place this as warm as possible upon the affected area and either change it when it cools down or cover the cloth with a sheet of plastic and place a hot water bottle on this. The heat will enhance the activity of the herb.

To make a poultice use either fresh or dried herbs. With the fresh plant you apply the bruised leaves or root material either directly on the skin or place it between thin gauze. With the dried herb, first make a paste by adding hot water, then apply in the same way as a compress.

## SAFETY

Herbalism is one of the oldest known ways of healing. The herbs we have suggested in this book have been used for centuries: they have passed the test of time, and are effective and often powerful. Although herbalism is a natural form of healing, this must not be confused with being entirely harmless. Herbs have a strong therapeutic value and they must be used with respect and common sense.

It is best to be cautious, and any problem that is severe or persists with the use of these herbs, should be taken to a qualified practitioner. It is unwise to continue using herbs over a prolonged period of time or to exceed a safe dose. As a general guide you can take an herb or herb mixture for six weeks, then have a break for two weeks before repeating for another six weeks if required. If in doubt consult a qualified herbalist.

It is always advisable to cross-reference any herb that you intend to use with an herbal reference book (see the Further Reading section).

## CHILDREN

For children aged 7-12 years halve the adult dosage. For children 2-6 years use a quarter. Only very mild herbs, e.g. Marshmallow and Chamomile should be used for infants under 2 years, and then use only 1-2 tablespoonfuls of infusion as a dose.

## PREGNANCY

All herbs should be specifically checked for their suitability during pregnancy. For a list of herbs to avoid see the entry under 'Pregnancy'.

## MEDICATION

Anyone taking prescribed medication should check with a qualified practitioner before taking medicinal herbs as drug-herb interactions are possible.

# HOMŒOPATHY

The word homœopathy comes from the Greek, it means 'similar suffering'. It is based on the law of similars: that 'like cures like'. A homœopathic remedy is chosen by matching the symptom picture of the patient with that of a remedy. For example, if a person is suffering from diarrhoea and vomiting, minute doses, in potentised form, of a remedy are given which in large, crude doses would cause vomiting and diarrhoea in a healthy person.

Homœopathic remedies do not work directly on the physical body, but rather, when the healing process is faulty, encourage the natural forces of the body to restore health and harmony. The correct homœopathic remedy will stimulate the person's vitality to send healing energy where it is needed, i.e. for physical, mental or emotional healing: thus, it is truly a holistic medicine.

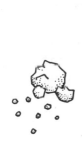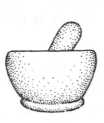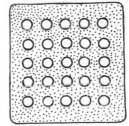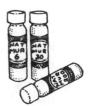

The remedies suggested in this book are for use in first-aid and acute situations only. If symptoms are severe, or persist, or are of a more chronic nature, a skilled homœopath should be consulted. If undergoing a course of homœopathic treatment from a practitioner, no other remedy should be taken without first consulting them about it. In many cases there is a 'miasmatic' background to an illness, i.e. an acquired or inherited disease tendency; and this can only be dealt with by constitutional treatment from a skilled practitioner.

## STORING AND TAKING
## HOMŒOPATHIC REMEDIES

Homœopathic remedies are very sensitive and should be stored in a dark, cool place, away from strong smells such as coffee, peppermint, camphor, eucalyptus and menthol. Similarly, those same substances should be avoided by the patient when taking a course of homœopathic treatment.

Homœopathic remedies should not be swallowed, but left to dissolve under the tongue. Food, drinks, smoking and toothpaste should be avoided for twenty minutes before and after taking a remedy.

Unless otherwise specified, remedies in the 6th potency should be taken one dose every three hours until there is some improvement, then dosage should be less frequent. Remedies in the 30th potency should be repeated once or twice a day, preferably at eight-hour intervals. Remedies in the 200th potency should be taken as a single dose, and not repeated unless otherwise directed. Remedies in any higher potency than the 200th should only be taken under the supervision of a qualified homœopath.

Once a homœopathic remedy has showed signs of working, and symptoms improve, then STOP taking the remedy. If the symptoms return some time after stopping taking the remedy, then repeat the remedy. Some illnesses may require more than one remedy to bring about a cure, the guideline is that if the symptoms change, then select a different remedy that covers the new picture.

# AROMATHERAPY

Aromatherapy is a form of treatment using essential oils. The term aromatherapy was first used by the French chemist Gattefosse. He researched into the medicinal properties of essential oils in the 1920s. Recorded history of the use of essential oils goes back to the time of the Ancient Egyptians who recognised the effects of fragrant plants, and discovered methods of extracting the oils from the plants to use in perfumes, cooking, ointments and salves and embalming their dead.

Each essential oil has its own therapeutic properties which have been proven by use through the ages, from the Ancient Egyptians, through to the Ancient Greeks, the Arabs, through China and India, and then brought to Europe. Today there is considerable scientific research being done on the properties of the various oils, but we believe that it is the subtle combinations of the components that constitute the whole oil that provides most benefit.

Essential oils are the essences obtained from flowers, leaves, barks, roots and berries by various methods of extraction. The method of extraction used varies according to the type of plant, and the part of the plant to be used. The quality of the oil will depend on the method of extraction and the quality of the plant. Major influences are the area where the plant was grown, and the weather during the growing season, which will be reflected in the price of the oil as with any crop.

Essential oils can be used to treat a wide range of ailments including first-aid, common minor ailments, stress-related diseases and skin problems. They are of great value in skin care, not just for cosmetic purposes, but also to aid such problems as acne, eczema, dermatitis, stretch marks and broken veins. Chemical copies of essential oil fragrances are used widely in commercial cosmetics and perfumery because they are much cheaper; but these will have none of the therapeutic properties of a pure essential oil, and may indeed be damaging if used in therapeutic doses. Check with your supplier that the oils you are going to purchase are pure and unadulterated, and not synthetic or blended oils.

An aromatherapist will use essential oils as part of a holistic programme of treatment. Diet, lifestyle, emotional stress, etc., will all be taken into consideration when choosing appropriate oils to suit the individual. Cleansing diets and exercises may be suggested throughout treatment to enhance healing and relaxation and promote the elimination of toxins. Whilst the oils that we suggest will be helpful to alleviate common and minor ailments, obviously this cannot replace the advice and treatment of a qualified aromatherapist where illness is more persistant or more severe.

## HOW TO APPLY ESSENTIAL OILS

### MASSAGE

Massage is one of the most successful and effective ways of employing the healing properties of essential oils. There are many good books and courses available today on massage. A regular light massage with essential oils will be beneficial to a person's well-being, and can be relaxing or stimulating depending on the oils chosen.

Before applying essential oils to the skin they must be diluted in a base oil. Suitable vegetable base oils are: almond, apricot kernel, avocado, grapeseed, olive, soya and wheatgerm. Of these, the light oils — almond, apricot kernel, grapeseed, soya — can be used on their own or combined. The heavier oils — avocado, olive, wheatgerm — will be rather strong smelling and sticky if used alone, and are better combined with one of the lighter oils, unless a very rich massage base is required.

The ratio of essential oil to base oil will vary according to the oil and the desired effect, but should fall within the range of one to three per cent of essential oil to base oil. Twenty drops of essential oil equals approximately 1 ml. This means that to 100 ml of base oil between twenty and sixty drops of essential oil (or of combined essential oils) will be added. If you wish to make up enough oil for only one massage then pour a little massage base oil onto a saucer and add just two or three drops of the required essential oil.

### INHALATIONS

Add three or four drops of the essential oil to a handkerchief, hold this near the nose every few moments to inhale the vapours.

Steam inhalations are very effective for colds, sore throats, coughs and congestion and for treating the skin of the face. To a bowl of steaming water add five to ten drops of essential oil, then place a towel over your head and the bowl and inhale the vapour for a few minutes. This can be repeated two or three times a day.

## BATHS

In a bath the penetration of the oils into the skin is aided by the heat of the water. Totally non-irritant essential oils such as chamomile, lavender and rose may be added directly to the bath (4-6 drops), all other oils should be pre-diluted in a little full-fat milk or base oil before adding to the bath so that no molecules of neat essential oil come into contact with sensitive mucous membranes. Add the essential-oil blend to the bath once it has been run and get in the water immediately, before the oils evaporate.

Foot or hand baths may be prepared in the same way using about five drops of essential oil to a bowl of hot water.

## COMPRESSES

Compresses can help a wide range of disorders. For a very small area e.g., a boil or insect sting, the essential oil can be used neat. Apply directly to the area and cover with a piece of cotton wool or warm, damp gauze.

For a larger area add ten drops of essential oil to 100 ml of hot water. Soak a piece of clean cotton or lint in the solution and place as hot as possible (without burning the skin) onto the affected area. To keep this warm, place a plastic bag over the cotton and hold a hot water bottle on it.

## SCENTING A ROOM

Add ten drops of essential oil to a plant spray containing water and spray in the room to purify the air after cooking, sickness, etc.

Aromatic burners can be purchased that use either a nightlight candle or an electric element to heat a plate that a few drops of the oil are placed on.

SAFETY

We do not recommend that essential oils are taken internally, although in certain circumstances specially qualified aromatherapists may prescribe this. Some essential oils that are not toxic externally are toxic internally.

Essential oils are highly concentrated substances and should always be treated with care and properly diluted before use. Some people may have an adverse reaction to a particular oil, so obviously its use should be discontinued in that case. Use common sense when dealing with these powerful, therapeutic substances.

Oils to be avoided during pregnancy are basil and sage.

Essential oils should never be used on babies. Only the mildest essential oils such as lavender, mandarin and chamomile should be used on children and always ensure oils are very well diluted before use on children, i.e. do not exceed a one per cent dilution.

Oils made from spices, e.g. cinnamon and clove and several of the citrus oils can irritate the skin, so do not use unless very well diluted.

# BACH FLOWER REMEDIES

The 38 remedies discovered by Dr Bach are made from a range of flowering plants and trees. The blooms are picked at their peak of condition, on a sunny day. They are prepared by very simple, natural means, which preserve their essence for use in the remedies. Flower remedies do not address specific illnesses or physical conditions, rather the personality, mood and emotional outlook of a person. They should be looked on as a way of restoring peace of mind, allowing the body to fight illness (whether mental or physical) by strengthening its own resources. They can be given quite safely to children or babies.

Dr Edward Bach MD, BS, DPH, MRCS, LRCP (1886-1936) trained and worked in conventional medicine in the early part of the last century.

His medical researches led him to the understanding that much of our ill-health originates in our emotional and mental state rather than in the physical body. Through intense study of the nature of plants he linked their qualities with certain states of being, chronic conditions and emotional states in people. He described a link between negative qualities in ourselves and the corresponding positive qualities in plants which can be used as remedies that bring hope to the desolate, strength to the exhausted and comfort to the distressed.

The Bach flower remedies work not by attacking disease but by flooding our bodies with the beautiful vibrations of our Higher Nature. They help to remake the contact with our true self, which has become hidden by our reaction to life's difficulties.

While the healing herbs of Dr Edward Bach will not interfere with other treatments, they do not replace professional advice if that is appropriate. They can be taken in any circumstances by anyone needing help.

## DIRECTIONS

Browse through the remedies using the list in the Appendix for any that you feel appropriate to you. It is usual to use a combination of remedies, limiting the number to no more than five or six. (Five Flower Remedy, if chosen, would count as one.)

Then dilute the mixture to dosage strength: put two drops from each chosen stock concentrate remedy into a small bottle of water (about 30 mls), adding a little brandy as a preservative if desired. If the Five Flower Remedy is chosen, then four drops of stock are used. Take four drops of the mixture, four times daily.

Alternatively, for short term problems, put two drops of each stock concentrate remedy into a glass of water and sip at intervals until there is relief.

Benefit comes from small quantity, regular use, rather than by the volume of remedy consumed. Don't worry that an inappropriate remedy might have an adverse reaction.

FIVE FLOWER REMEDY

The combination that Dr Bach called the 'rescue remedy' has become the most widely used flower remedy. It is a mix of five different flower essences which together help deal with any emergency or stressful event. Use it when taking an exam or driving test, having to speak in front of a crowd, going to a job interview, after some kind of accident or even argument with a loved one - there are countless times when five flower remedy comes in useful.

Many people carry this remedy in their car, briefcase or handbag, just to have it ready should it be needed. Many pet owners also find this remedy beneficial for stress in animals, such as a visit to the vet, or fear of being left alone.

The information above, and the list in the Appendix, have been provided by

Healing Herbs of Dr Bach,
PO Box 65,
Hereford,
HR2 0DX
www.healingherbs.co.uk

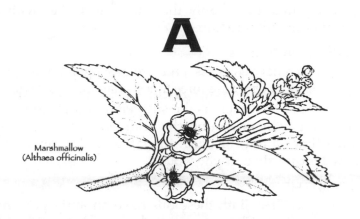

Marshmallow
(Althaea officinalis)

## ABRASIONS

A graze is an injury caused by scraping or rubbing. The important thing is to carefully cleanse the area using an antiseptic lotion to prevent infection. A clean, dry dressing may be applied to keep the area protected, this must be changed regularly.

HERBS

*Comfrey, Golden Seal, Marigold, St John's Wort:* To promote healing and prevent infection. Combine or use separately. Make an infusion to use as an antiseptic wash, or make a poultice.

TINCTURES

*Marigold:* Promotes healing.

*St John's Wort:* Antiseptic and pain relieving.

You may be able to purchase the above as a mixture referred to as *Hypericum and Calendula*.

Dilute four or five drops of the tincture in a little cool, boiled water and bathe the area.

OINTMENTS

*Marigold:* Promotes healing.

You may be able to purchase the above combined in an ointment referred to as *Hypericum and Calendula Ointment*.

Clean the area, then apply the ointment. Cover with a piece of clean lint if required.

## HOMŒOPATHY

*Arnica 6:* To relieve soreness, promote healing and help prevent infection. One dose three times a day for two days.

*Ferrum Phos 6X:* If there is the suspicion of infection, e.g. heat and redness around the abrased area. One dose three times a day, or crush the tablet and sprinkle the powder directly onto the wound.

## AROMATHERAPY

*Lavender, Tea Tree:* Both these oils have an antiseptic and healing effect. Choose one of them and sprinkle 2-3 drops onto the affected area.

# ABSCESS

An encapsulated collection of pus. If this becomes inflamed there will be heat, redness and throbbing present.

Anyone who is prone to such infection could benefit from a cleansing diet as well as the following suggestions. Garlic capsules will be a useful dietary supplement. If the patient develops a generalised temperature, or the symptoms are persistent, then professional advice must be immediately.

## HERBS

### EXTERNAL

*Chickweed, Comfrey, Marshmallow Root, Plantain, Slippery Elm:* Combine or use separately. Make a poultice to draw out the poisons.

### INTERNAL

*Burdock Root, Cleavers, Echinacea, Golden Seal, Yellow Dock:* Combine and make a decoction using one teaspoonful per cup of water, or use tinctures. Drink a cupful three times a day for ten days to prevent the infection spreading and eliminate the toxins.

HOMŒOPATHY

*Apis 30:* Every four hours when there is swelling with stinging pains; there may also be redness and throbbing.

*Belladonna 30:* Every four hours for a threatening abscess with redness pain and throbbing. The part feels hot to touch.

*Calc Sulph 6X:* Three times a day if the discharge continues too long and the wound is slow to heal.

*Hepar Sulph 30:* Three times a day when the pus is forming and it needs to be discharged. The area is very painful and aggravated by touch.

*Silica 30:* Three times a day when the pus has formed but the poison is slow to come away. Assists suppuration.

AROMATHERAPY

*Chamomile, Lavender:* Use externally, making a compress with the essential oils.


# ACCIDENTS

Most accidents are minor and can be dealt with by using one of the remedies suggested. For more serious accidents, call emergency services and give *Arnica* or *Five Flower Remedy* while waiting. If there is any loss of consciousness or excessive bleeding, seek professional help immediately. (See also: ABRASIONS, BRUISES, BURNS, EYE INJURIES, FRACTURES, SHOCK, SPRAINS and STRAINS.)

HERBS

*Balm, Chamomile, Skullcap:* For shock and stress. Combine or use separately to make a calming infusion. Drink a cupful every few hours as necessary.

HOMŒOPATHY

*Arnica* for shock and trauma. Reduces pain and bruising and will help prevent haemorrhage.

*Arnica 6 or 30:* For minor accidents. Take three doses of the 6th potency a day for five days, or one dose of the 30th potency for three days.

*Arnica 200:* For more severe accidents. Two doses eight hours apart.

*Arnica Ointment:* This may be applied locally (not for broken skin).

## AROMATHERAPY

*Eucalyptus, Geranium, Lavender, Tea Tree:* These are pain relieving and healing. Apply externally to the affected area.

## BACH FLOWER REMEDIES

*Five Flower Remedy:* For shock and trauma. Take a few drops internally or apply externally.

*Five Flower Cream:* Apply externally.


# ACNE

A skin complaint occuring particularly among adolescents. Often this is a result of hormonally induced hyperactivity of the oil-producing glands and is characterised by blackheads and pustules, usually on the face and back.

There is a dietary factor to this condition which is related to the body's ability to metabolise fats and carbohydrates. The intake of fats, sweets and carbohydrates must be reduced and replaced with more fresh fruits and vegetables. Many sufferers also benefit from eliminating milk from their diet as milk can aggravate the inflammatory process.

## HERBS

### INTERNAL

*Burdock, Cleavers, Dandelion, Echinacea, Red Clover, Yellow Dock:* Combine the herbs and make an infusion using one teaspoon of herbs to one cup of boiling water, or use the tinctures. Take three times a day for at least three weeks. This will help cleanse the system and clear the skin.

EXTERNAL

*Chickweed, Elderflower, Marigold:* Combine in equal parts and use as a facial steam.

HOMŒOPATHY

For persistent or severe acne constitutional treatment by a qualified practitioner will be necessary.

*Silica, Sulphur, Carbo Veg 6:* Cleans out the system, good for unhealthly skin. One three times a day for four days, then two weeks later repeat for four days.

*Calc Sulph 6X:* For pimples and pustules with a yellow discharge. One twice a day for two weeks.

AROMATHERAPY

FACIAL STEAM

*Chamomile, Juniper, Lavender, Palmarosa:* Add one drop of each oil to hot water and use as a facial steam. Use two or three times a week after cleansing.

FACIAL OILS

*Bergamot, Cedarwood, Chamomile, Geranium, Lavender, Palmarosa:* Dilute in a suitable vegetable oil base a few drops of the essential oils. Massage into the skin morning and evening after cleansing.


# AGEING

A natural process causing a slowing down of cell division.

Probably the most important factors to consider regarding ageing are diet, environment and stress. A wholefood diet, with plenty of fresh fruit and vegetables is vital to provide the right balance of vitamins and minerals necessary for youthfulness. Antioxidants in particular help to slow down the deterioration of cells. Many herbs and fresh foods are naturally rich in antioxidants, or you can take an antioxidant supplement.

The ability to cope with or even enjoy the ageing process depends on the lifestyle one adopts. Excessive stress is always ageing and can be rapidly so. Regular exercise is essential and meditation is helpful. Professional counselling can be beneficial to help an individual isolate the particular factors in their lifestyle that could be changed to their long-term benefit. The following suggestions may be a useful adjunct to considering appropriate changes in lifestyle. (See also: WRINKLES.)

## HERBS
*Ginseng:* This was traditionally used in China to promote longevity, aid memory and for its stimulant properties. A course of *Ginseng* may be taken in a variety of forms, e.g. root, tincture or tablets, for up to six weeks of each year. *Ginseng* is not suitable if you suffer with hypertension — in which case consult a qualified herbalist.

## HOMŒOPATHY
*Calc Phos 6X:* Stimulates healthy cell division. Good for exhaustion and for convalescence. Take one dose morning and evening for ten days.

## AROMATHERAPY
*Lavender:* Promotes healthy cell division. Use externally as a massage after diluting in a suitable vegetable oil base. Alternatively add a couple of drops to a warm bath or use as a facial steam.

*Neroli, Frankincense, Rose, Sandalwood:* A useful combination for ageing skin. Add a few drops of each oil to a suitable vegetable oil base and use as a massage oil. Or combine the oils and use a few drops in a facial steam.

*Wheatgerm Oil:* This vegetable oil is naturally rich in vitamin E which is said to slow down the ageing process by keeping cells healthy and well oxygenated. Use 10% of *Wheatgerm Oil* in a lighter massage base oil such as *Almond Oil.*

*Rosehip Seed Oil:* This oil is very rich in essential fatty acids and is a specific oil for repairing scarred or sun damaged skin, it will help to slow down the signs of ageing.

## ALCOHOLISM

Professional advice should be sought to deal with the physiological and psychological problems related to a dependence on alcohol. One of the most common physical ailments resulting from an excessive intake of alcohol is liver disease. (See also: LIVER PROBLEMS.) The following suggestions are meant to supplement, not replace, professional help.

### HERBS

*Passiflora, Skullcup, Valerian:* A tea made from a combination of these herbs will be calming to the nervous system and helpful for withdrawal symptoms including delerium tremens. One cupful three times a day.

*Milk Thistle:* Helps repair damage to the liver caused by alcohol abuse. Use half a teaspoon to a cupful of boiling water, infuse for fifteen minutes and drink three times a day. Or use the capsules.

### HOMŒOPATHY

Individual consultation is recommended.

### AROMATHERAPY

A course of treatment by a qualified aromatherapist would be of help to provide support.

### BACH FLOWER REMEDIES

The emotional states leading to a dependence on alcohol are varied. Seek advice or refer to more detailed books on the Bach flower remedies.

## ALLERGIES

Allergic reactions are caused when the antigen production of the liver, pancreas and spleen exceed the normal production. Various natural or artificial substances can trigger this response. The most commonly experienced symptoms are irritation of the mucous membranes and skin. A wide range of other symptoms, including behavioural ones, are the subject of extensive recent research.

There are two approaches to the treatment of allergies. One is to isolate the irritating agent and then avoid it, the other is to treat the individual constitutionally until they have a healthier vitality and no longer produce the symptoms of allergy. Professional advice is suggested.

(See also: HAYFEVER.)

### HERBS

*Chamomile, Yarrow:* These herbs will soothe an allergic response. Drink a cupful of the infusion as necessary.

*Nettle:* This herb is a specific for reducing allergies. Drink a cupful three times a day for a month. Infuse one heaped teaspoon of the herbs to a cupful of boiling water for ten minutes.

### HOMŒOPATHY

*Apis 30:* Skin allergies with swelling and burning, stinging pains. One three times a day for up to five days.

*Ferrum Phos 6X:* Will alleviate inflammation or irritation caused by an allergic reaction. One three times a day for up to ten days.

*Urtica Urens 30:* For alleviation of urticaria, a result of some allergies. One three times a day for up to five days.

### AROMATHERAPY

*Chamomile, Lavender, Yarrow:* Apply in a massage oil base for local skin irritation.

BACH FLOWER REMEDIES
*Five Flower Cream:* Apply locally to affected area. Good for
  local skin irritation.


# ANÆMIA

Diminished oxygen-carrying capacity of the blood, due to
a reduction in the numbers of red cells or in their content
of haemoglobin, or both. The cause may be inadequate
production of red cells or excessive or prolonged loss
of blood. Even a small amount of blood loss over a prolonged period of time may cause anæmia, e.g. from an
internal ulcer, so persistent anæmia should always be
referred to a practitioner for precise diagnosis.

Many women are considered to be anæmic due to an inability to assimilate iron at a rate sufficient to make up for
that lost in the blood during the menstrual cycle.

Laxatives will cause a loss of iron from the body, and con-
tinual drinking of coffee and tea will retard the absorption
of the mineral iron. Many drugs will also cause anæmia.

The mineral iron is essential for the formation of red
blood cells. Foods naturally rich in iron include: meat,
eggs, lentils, apricots, green-leaf vegetables, molasses and
beetroot.

The minerals calcium and copper, vitamin C and the B
group vitamins must also be present for the body to be
able to assimilate iron. A balanced diet of natural foods
may supply sufficient quantities of these vitamins and
minerals, otherwise food supplements may be taken, and
vegetarians in particular may require additional vitamin
B12. Floradix is a particularly useful iron supplement.

HERBS
*Alfalfa, Centaury, Dandelion Root, Nettle, Rosehip, Watercress:*
  Combine and make an infusion using one teaspoon of
  herbs to a cup of boiling water. Drink a cupful three
  times a day for a month to six weeks.

23

## HOMŒOPATHY

For chronic cases, a qualified homœopath should be consulted.

*Ferrum Phos 6X:* This tissue salt will enable the body to assimilate iron and use it more efficiently. Take one three times a day for a month.

## BACH FLOWER REMEDIES

*Olive:* This will help with the exhaustion and weariness often associated with anæmia.

# ANXIETY

A feeling of uneasiness and apprehension accompanied with tension which may or may not have an obvious cause. Anxiety may be associated with tight breathing, palpitations and perspiration.

Continued anxiety can cause illness such as digestive disorders, headaches, backache, high blood pressure and many other troubles.

Counselling may be needed to help the person redirect their fears and understand their symptoms. A professional practitioner should be consulted if the anxiety is extreme.

Diet, as always, has an important role to play. Check especially that your diet contains sufficient calcium and magnesium, and vitamins B and C.

## HERBS

*Balm, Chamomile, Lime Flowers, Orange Blossom, Passiflora, Scullcap, Valerian, Vervain:* These are all relaxing nerve tonics. They will soothe stress and relieve feelings of anxiety and panic. Combine and drink a cupful of infusion, or use the tinctures, three times a day.

## HOMŒOPATHY

*AAA 30 (Ambra Grisea, Anacardium, Arg Nit):* Anxiety prior to a particular" event, e.g. aeroplane flight, interview, exam, etc. Take one dose each night for a week before the event and one dose on the day.

*Aconite 30:* Anxiety dating from a fright, shock or accident. Panic attacks. Fear will die any minute. One dose twice a day for two or three days.

*Arg Nit 30:* Anticipatory diarrhoea. Stage fright, etc. One or two doses.

*Calc Phos, Kali Phos, Mag Phos 6X:* Nervous fatigue. Calms down after stress and strain. Results of work pressure. Stress headaches. Inability to relax. One three times a day for ten days or when necessary.

*Ignatia 200:* Anxiety dating from a particular disappointment, shock, bereavement, etc. One dose only.

*Kali Phos 6X:* Nervousness, sleeplessness, weariness, tension. For nerves 'on edge'. One three times a day for ten days.

*Mag Phos 6X:* Nervous tension and tense muscles causing cramps, headaches, trembling, etc. One three times a day for ten days.

AROMATHERAPY

*Geranium, Lavender, Melissa, Ylang Ylang:* Dilute in a bath oil base and add to a bath, or combine two or three and dilute in a suitable base massage oil for a calming massage. As a soothing fragrance *Basil* and *Clary Sage* could also be used on an aromatic burner.

BACH FLOWER REMEDIES

Choose from among the following and refer to a more detailed book to see if there are indications for other Bach flower remedies.

*Five Flower Remedy:* Apprehension, shock, anguish, panic attacks, etc.

*Agrimony:* For those who suffer anxiety but pretend to be happy and cheerful.

*Aspen:* Vague anxiety, apprehensions and fears of unknown origin.

*Cherry Plum:* Desperation, fear of mental collapse.

*Mimulus:* Fear and apprehension of known events.

*Red Chestnut:* Anxiety about others, e.g. members of one's family.

*Rock Rose:* Extreme anxiety, panic.

*White Chestnut:* Persistent anxious thoughts. Preoccupation with some worry.

# APHRODISIACS

A substance that increases sexual desire and improves sexual potency.

## HERBS

### FOR MEN

*Ashwaganda, Damiana, Ginseng, Saw Palmetto:* These are tonics for the male reproductive system; traditionally used as sexual stimulants. Combine the tinctures and take three times daily for up to six weeks. *Ginseng* is not suitable if you suffer from hypertension.

### FOR WOMEN

*Chinese Angelica, Damiana, Schizandra:* Hormonal tonics and sexual stimulants for women. Combine tinctures and take three times daily for up to six weeks.

## HOMŒOPATHY

Constitutional treatment to build up the vitality is recommended.

## AROMATHERAPY

*Cedarwood, Coriander, Jasmine, Patchouli, Rose, Vetiver, Ylang Ylang:* Combine two or three of these essential oils and mix into a vegetable base oil for a sexually stimulating massage, or add two or three drops of one of the essential oils to a warm bath. Alternatively, a few drops of one of the oils burnt in an essential oil burner will create a suitably relaxing atmosphere. Suitable for men and women.

## APPETITE LOSS

The appetite can be a good indicator of the general state of health. Chronic appetite loss should be referred to a practitioner.

The remedies suggested here will be useful in the recovery phase of an illness such as influenza.

(See also: CONVALESCENCE.)

### HERBS

*Centaury, Fennel:* These 'bitter' herbs will stimulate the appetite. Combine the herbs and make an infusion, drink three times a day. A pinch of powdered *Cinnamon* may be added. Alternatively take in tincture form.

### HOMŒOPATHY

*Calc Phos 6X:* Assists digestion and assimilation of food. Good for convalescence, may help stimulate the appetite. Take one twice a day for ten days.

### AROMATHERAPY

*Bergamot, Coriander, Fennel, Juniper:* Dilute in a vegetable base oil and rub into the stomach area twice daily to help stimulate the appetite.


## ARTHRITIS

Inflammation of a joint, causing pain and leading to restriction of movement. A holistic style practitioner should be consulted because it is essential to treat the whole being; otherwise healing will be only slight or temporary. Factors that need to be investigated are: the genetic framework, environmental factors — diet, stress, injury — and also the pyschological contribution.

The most common forms of this disease are osteo-arthritis and rheumatoid arthritis.

Again, it must be stressed that professional guidance is essential; the following suggestions may provide some relief whilst professional help is being sought.

Acupuncture and naturopathy are particularly recommended for this complaint.

(See also: GOUT, RHEUMATISM.)

## HERBS

*Celery Seed, Devil's Claw, Feverfew, Meadowsweet, Prickly Ash, White Willow:* A mixture to clear uric acid and toxins, reduce inflammation and relieve pain. Add *Bogbean* if the symptoms are worse in damp weather. Combine the herbs and make a decoction to drink, or use the tinctures, three times daily for one month to six weeks.

A poultice for swollen joints that are relieved by warmth may be made from nine parts of *Slippery Elm* to one part of *Cayenne*. Add 75 g of the mixture to hot water to make a paste. Spread onto a cloth and apply to the affected area. Leave on for as long as possible.

Alternatively, for joints that are relieved by cool, a cabbage poultice will be helpful.

## HOMŒOPATHY

Constitutional treatment will be of most benefit. The following may assist while alternative treatment is being considered.

*Ferrum Phos 6X:* In acute attacks with inflammation of the joint. One three times a day for up to ten days.

*Nat Phos 6X:* Will help clear out uric acid. One twice a day for ten days.

## AROMATHERAPY

*Chamomile, Eucalyptus, Juniper, Lavender, Lemon:* Combine and dilute in almond oil, massage into the afflicted joint and wrap in a warm cover. Or add a few drops of the chosen essential oil or oils to a warm bath.

## FOOD SUPPLEMENTS

*Cod Liver Oil or Flax Seed Oil:* Oils rich in essential fatty acids have been found to help many sufferers.

## ASTHMA

Asthma can be defined as a difficulty in breathing caused by muscular spasm. The spasm makes it difficult to cough away mucus which collects in the small bronchi thus further impeding breathing.

There is a hereditary factor to asthma, and other causes include allergy, infection and emotional disturbance. Treatment of asthma is a difficult, complicated problem and should be handled by a qualified practitioner. In particular, the assessment of the severity of acute episodes calls for considerable experience.

A diet eliminating all mucous-stimulating foods (e.g. dairy products) may be of help.

The switch over from orthodox inhalers and medication should not be attempted unless under the supervision of a suitably qualified practitioner. The following suggestions may offer some relief whilst such professional help is being sought.

### HERBS

*Coltsfoot, Elecampane, Hyssop, Liquorice, Mullein, Plantain, Wild Cherry Bark:* An expectorant mixture to help clear mucus and tonify the lungs. Mix in equal parts. Infuse one teaspoonful of herbs to a cupful of boiling water for ten minutes or use the tinctures. Take three times a day for up to a month.

*Motherwort, Scullcap:* A soothing and calming mixture to drink after a spasm attack. Combine and drink a cupful of the infusion every couple of hours.

### HOMŒOPATHY

Constitutional treatment by a qualified practitioner can be of great benefit to asthma sufferers.

*Mag Phos 6X:* May help to relax spasms. Take one dose every two hours during an attack, or one dose three times a day for ten days as a longer-term course.

AROMATHERAPY

*Chamomile, Eucalyptus, Frankincense, Lavender:* Combine and add to a base oil for a relaxing and decongestant massage. Or add a few drops to an essential oil burner and place nearby.

BACH FLOWER REMEDIES

*Five Flower Remedy:* Add a few drops to a little water and sip as often as required to alleviate fear and panic.

# ATHLETE'S FOOT

A fungal infection of the skin, usually found between the toes.

Keep the feet clean and dry. Wear only natural fibres for socks and shoes. If the toes are pushed together place a small piece of cotton wool between them so that air can circulate and moisture is not retained.

HERBS

*Burdock, Echinacea, Thyme, Yellow Dock:* Combine and make an infusion to drink three times a day for at least two weeks.

*Marigold, Myrrh, Thyme:* Combine the tinctures or make an infusion to bathe the affected part three times a day.

HOMŒOPATHY

*Nat Phos, Nat Sulph, Silica 6X:* For fungal infections. One three times a day for ten days.

AROMATHERAPY

*Eucalyptus, Lavender, Thyme:* Combine the above oils and make a strong dilution in a vegetable oil base. Massage a couple of drops of the oil into the affected area twice a day after bathing.

*Tea Tree:* Apply directly to the affected area.

# B

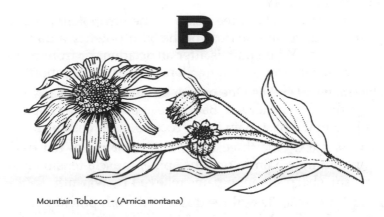

Mountain Tobacco - (Arnica montana)

## BACKACHE

Pains in the back are experienced by many people and the causes are very varied. Bad posture caused by tension will create strained muscles resulting in pain. We would advise the Alexander Technique to correct this. Pain in the back at the level of the waist may be due to spinal disease, or kidney and bladder infections; various toxins otherwise eliminated through the kidney and bladder are deposited in surrounding tissue areas, especially the spinal joints of the lumbar region. Low back pain may be due to a disorder of the reproductive organs in women. Much back pain is the result of overstraining or injury. If the vertebra or pelvis is out of alignment, a manipulative therapy such as Osteopathy or Chiropractice should be considered. A diagnosis to rule out a more serious causative factor is vital: full examination, X-rays, or other investigations may be indicated.

### HERBS

*Balm, Scullcap, Vervain, White Willow:* These are antispasmodic and pain-relieving herbs to reduce inflammation and relieve pain. Combine and infuse one teaspoon of equal parts of the herbs or use the tinctures and take three times a day.

*Comfrey Oil:* Massage daily.

31

## HOMŒOPATHY

*Arnica 6 or 30:* Take three doses of the 6th potency a day for five days, or one dose of the 30th potency a day for three days. When pain is after an accident or from over-exertion such as gardening, dancing or playing sports.

*Hypericum 30 or 200:* One or two doses for injuries involving the spinal nerves. Backache resulting from spinal injury in the past, pain in the coccycx after childbirth.

*Mag Phos 6X:* One three times a day for up to ten days for neuralgic pains along the spine, muscle tension and spasm, sharp shooting pains relieved by warmth.

*Rhus Tox 6 or 30:* Take three doses of the 6th potency twice a day for five days, or one dose of the 30th potency for three days. For muscular stiffness due to over-exertion or from exposure to cold and damp.

## AROMATHERAPY

*Ginger, Juniper, Lavender, Marjoram, Rosemary:* For a soothing and warming massage. Combine five drops of each in a light vegetable oil base and massage over the painful area.

# BED WETTING

This is not usually considered a problem until the child reaches school age. It is very often hereditary, and sometimes caused by an organic problem, so it is advisable to take the child to a physician for an examination. There is nearly always a psychological factor to take into account. Prolonged bed wetting causes stress to the child and to the parents, so it must be treated with care and understanding. A non-stimulating diet should be encouraged cutting out soft drinks, white sugar, and food colourings, especially orange. (See also: INCONTINENCE.)

## HERBS

*Catnip, Chamomile, Horsetail, St John's Wort:* Use one teaspoon to a cup and sweeten with a little honey so the child will drink it. Try two cups a day.

## HOMŒOPATHY

There are numerous remedies to help in this situation and it is important to find the correct remedy that fits the nature of the child, so if the pattern persists or the child suddenly starts wetting the bed, go and see a homœopath.

## BACH FLOWER REMEDIES

Look at the remedies covering fears and anxiety and decide if your child could be helped by them. (See the list in the Appendix and cross-reference with more detailed books mentioned in the Further Reading.)

# BITES AND STINGS

Some people are more sensitive than others to bites. If symptoms of collapse or difficulty in breathing develop, emergency professional treatment must be sought. The following remedies will help deal with the pain, sting or shock; but it is also important to employ methods to stop infection developing.

## HERBS

*Witchazel:* Will relieve heat and inflammation. Make an infusion or use distilled *Witchazel* and apply externally.

*Marigold, St John's Wort:* If the skin is broken, to prevent infection and promote healing. Make an infusion or use tinctures and apply externally at regular intervals. To prevent a bite becoming infected take *Echinacea* decoction or tincture internally. Crushed *Garlic* or a slice of raw *Onion* applied externally may relieve stinging and reduce risk of infection.

*Lavender, Pennyroyal, Pyrethrum, Southernwood, Tansy, Wormwood:* For repelling insects. Make an infusion from the above herbs and apply to the skin (when cool), or spray in a room.

## HOMŒOPATHY

*Apis 30:* Wasp or bee stings, swelling, redness, stinging, smarting pains, worse for heat. Symptoms of collapse. One every few hours until improvement occurs.

*Arnica 30:* Bites from mammals where bruising is marked and shock is present. One or two doses.

*Caladium 6 or 30:* Mosquito bites. Two or three times a day as necessary.

*Hypericum 30:* Punctured skin by bites or stings; skin tingling, burning pains radiating from injury. One or two doses.

*Lachesis 30:* Bites from poisonous animals, e.g. snakes, spiders. Part looks purple or blue. This is only a temporary measure on your way to the emergency room at the hospital.

*Ledum 30:* Punctured wounds, dog or insect bites. Oedematous swelling, bruising, parts can become red and inflamed. Bites may become infected. Try this remedy first for horsefly, wasp and dog bites. One dose as often as needed.

## AROMATHERAPY

*Citronella, Eucalyptus, Peppermint:* Use diluted in vegetable oil as a repellent, apply to exposed areas. We recommend also that these oils can be burned in the room to deter insects.

*Eucalyptus, Lavender, Melissa:* After-sting care. Dab any of these oils on the affected area.

*Tea Tree:* This can be used neat as a repellent and to relieve a bite or sting.

## BACH FLOWER REMEDIES

*Five Flower Remedy:* To soothe the patient and help with shock. Take a few drops internally or apply externally.

*Five Flower Cream:* Apply locally to soothe the bite or sting.

# BOILS

A boil is a painful, acute inflammation around the root of a hair.

Boils must not be squeezed as this would cause infection to spread. Boils are a symptom that the body contains waste and toxic matter, so a cleansing diet is recommended along with appropriate treatment.

## HERBS

*Marshmallow, Slippery Elm:* Use either herb as a poultice to help draw pus from the boil.

*Echinacea, Burdock Root, Dandelion Leaf:* A blood purifying combination. Combine in equal parts and make a decoction using a heaped teaspoon of herbs to a mug of water and simmer for ten minutes. Strain and drink a cupful three times a day for ten days. These herbs may also be taken as tinctures.

## HOMŒOPATHY

*Arnica 30:* A crop of small, painful boils. One dose three times a day for five days.

*Belladonna 30:* The boil is beginning to form. Heat, throbbing pain and redness are present. One dose three times a day for three days.

*Silica 30:* For boils where the pus has formed but healing has come to a standstill. One dose three times a day for up to five days.

*Tarentula 30:* Boils that are very painful and inflamed: intense itching and burning pains. One dose three times a day for up to five days.

## AROMATHERAPY

*Chamomile, Lavender, Lemon, Thyme:* Any of the above may be used. Add two or three drops to half a cupful of warm water; dip in a piece of cotton wool and apply this to the boil. Repeat two or three times a day.

## BREAST FEEDING

All indications suggest that the breast-fed child will be healthier; the colostrum produced after childbirth contains antibodies which give protection against infections. This early protection fills the immunity gap and so babies fed on breast milk are more resistant to infections than those fed by bottled milk. Putting the baby to the breast as soon as the cord is cut encourages the flow of milk, gives comfort to the baby and forms an early bond with the mother. Breast feeding is usually on demand, which means it is going to be draining for the mother, so plenty of rest is needed between feeds. Small regular meals and an increase in fluids are needed to help maintain a flow of milk, avoid over-spiced foods, garlic and acid fruits which might cause colic in the baby.

(See also: MASTITIS.)

HERBS

*Aniseed, Caraway, Dill, Fennel, Fenugreek, Holy thistle:* Any of these herbs will help to maintain sufficient supply of milk. Choose one and infuse one teaspoon to a cupful of boiling water, and drink two or three times daily.

*Alfalfa* is rich in minerals and *Vervain* is soothing, so these can also be drunk when needed as an infusion.

*Marigold Tincture:* For cracked painful nipples, bathe with ten drops diluted in warm water. May also be applied as a cream.

If it becomes necessary to dry up the milk, drink an infusion of *Sage* three times a day.

HOMŒOPATHY

*Calc Phos 6X:* Three times a day for maintaining general health. Exhaustion.

*Causticum 30:* Three times a day for up to five days for cracked nipples and poor milk flow.

*China 6:* Twice daily for exhaustion brought on by breast feeding. Take for ten days.

*Silica 30:* Three times a day for two days if there is any sign of abscess forming on the nipple, reducing the flow of milk. These homœopathic suggestions can be tried, but do consult a homœopath if the symptoms persist for longer than two days.

## AROMATHERAPY
*Rose:* For sore nipples; massage with a couple of drops of Rose oil in a little almond oil base. Wash before feeding, as any essential oils are too strong for the baby.

*Geranium, Lavender, Rose:* For inflammation of the breast, dilute one drop of each in a pint of cold water and use as a compress. However, if the condition persists, consult a practitioner.

## BACH FLOWER REMEDIES
*Olive:* This might be useful for the extreme exhaustion felt by some nursing mothers.

## BRONCHITIS
Acute bronchitis is a common condition involving inflammation and infection of the respiratory tract. It is common in the winter months and particularly in the elderly, the frail and those with a chronic chest disorder. Acute bronchitis often occurs in children with infectious fevers, especially measles, influenza and whooping cough. Symptoms are those of a mild fever with a cough, possibly pain beneath the sternum and breathing is usually a little faster than normal. The condition usually subsides in a few days with rest in bed, and is serious only in young children and elderly people where inflammation may spread and cause broncho-pneumonia. Repeated attacks may give rise to chronic bronchitis.

In chronic bronchitis there is swelling and thickening of the lining of the bronchial tree and obstruction to air entry is made worse by the presence of thick mucus. This can cause a serious debility, and must be dealt with by an experienced practitioner. Cigarette smoking, air pollution by smoke and sulphur dioxide, or working in a dusty atmosphere may be contributing causes.

Chronic bronchitis must be referred to a practitioner for constitutional treatment. The following remedies may be tried for the early stages of acute bronchitis, but in young children or if the symptoms persist then professional help should be sought.

## HERBS

*Coltsfoot, Elecampane, Hyssop, Iceland Moss, Mullein, Thyme:* These herbs combine an antimicrobial and expectorant effect with a demulcent action, soothing the inflamed tissues. Combine and infuse one teaspoon to a cup three times a day. Or exclude the Icelandic Moss and use the tinctures.

## HOMŒOPATHY

*Aconite 6 or 30:* Take three doses of the 6th potency a day for five days, or one dose of the 30th potency a day for three days. When cough comes on suddenly after exposure to cold winds, beginning of a fever, short dry cough which wakes the patient from sleep, patient is frightened and restless.

*Ant Tart 6 or 30:* Two or three doses for three or four days, patient is pale with a cold sweat, rattling cough with much mucous in the chest but less and less is raised as the patient becomes weaker. Coated tongue, averse to food and drink.

*Ars Alb 6 or 30:* Two or three doses for three or four days, suffocative cough, great tightness felt in the chest. Patient is anxious and restless, chilly patient. Desires sips of hot drinks.

*Belladonna 6 or 30:* Two or three doses for two or three days, for spasmodic cough with fever. Patient is delirious and has a high fever.

*Bryonia 6 or 30:* Two or three doses a day for three or four days for hard, dry, barking cough. Chest is painful and patient holds it when coughing, cough worse at night and from eating and drinking. Very irritable patient who wants to be left alone. Thirsty.

*Causticum 6 or 30:* Two or three doses for three or four days for a hard, scraping cough which hurts the chest. Any mucus slips back down before it can be cleared.

*Ferrum Phos 6X:* Three times a day for three or four days for the first signs of fever and inflammation. Short, acute, painful coughs. Try this first and hopefully other remedies won't be needed if you act fast enough.

*Ipecac 6 or 30:* Two or three doses over two or three days when the cough is preceeded by vomiting or mucus causes vomiting. Useful in children who cannot raise the mucus by coughing, but do vomit it up.

*Phosphorus 6 or 30:* Two or three doses for three or four days with a very irritating, tormenting cough, thirst for ice cold drinks, patient is shaking and weak, fearful and does not want to be left alone.

*Pulsatilla 6 or 30:* Two or three doses over three or four days with a catarrhal condition which descends to the chest; may follow on from measles. Thick yellow-green catarrh, tightness in chest, desires fresh air, dry cough worse at night.

*Sulphur 30:* Two or three doses eight hours apart when there is a sensation of weight on the chest, unpleasant smelling sweat, waves of heat and cold, patient is weary and not responding well to treatment, red orifices.

AROMATHERAPY

*Benzoin, Eucalyptus, Thyme:* Inhale steam from a bowl of hot water into which two or three drops of the essential oil has been put, or dilute in a vegetable base oil to massage onto the chest area.

## BRUISES

A bruise is the result of a blow or fall causing damage to the soft tissue beneath the skin, breaking the skin capillaries. As the blood clots the bruise becomes discoloured.

### HERBS

*Comfrey, Marigold, Witchazel, Yarrow:* Make an infusion using one tablespoon of each to a pint of water and use as a compress over the injured area.

*Arnica Ointment:* This is the most effective remedy for bruises but do not use if the skin is broken.

*Arnica Tincture:* This can also be used. Apply externally.

*Witchazel distilled:* Dab on locally with cotton wool.

### HOMŒOPATHY

*Arnica 30:* Take one three times a day to help the bruising and to counteract any effects of shock. Take for two days.

*Hypericum 30:* Two doses where bruising is very painful and relieved by warmth.

*Ledum 30:* Two doses when bruising becomes black or swollen, e.g. black eyes.

*Ruta 30:* Two doses for painful bruising of the bones e.g. shin.

### AROMATHERAPY

*Lavender:* Apply locally over bruised area.

*Helichrysum, Marjoram:* Dilute in cold water and use as a compress.

## BURNS

Treatment obviously depends on the severity of the burn; minor burns and scalds can be dealt with safely at home, more serious burns should be admitted to casualty, without attempting to remove clothing, etc., which may further damage the skin. Internal treatment for shock, e.g. *Five Flower Remedy* may safely be given. Chemical burns must be washed with cold running water for at least five minutes. If blisters form do not puncture as they form a protective cushion to the damaged area.

## HERBS

*Aloe Vera:* An excellent remedy for burns, including sunburn. Grow a plant in the kitchen, break off a leaf and squeeze out the gel on the burn. It is also available commercially as an ointment or gel.

*Comfrey, Marigold, St John's Wort:* Make an infusion from any of the above and bathe the burn to help promote healing. *St John's Wort Oil* may also be applied using cotton wool to relieve pain and promote healing.

## TINCTURES

When using tinctures to treat burns add a teaspoonful of tincture to a cupful of cool, boiled water. Soak a pad of gauze in this lotion, which must be large enough to cover the burn, apply the gauze, cover with lint and bandage. Remove the lint whenever the dressing feels dry and re-soak the gauze by moistening it with a few drops of the lotion, this prevents any tearing of the new skin cells and allows undisturbed growth to take place under cover of the dressing. Once a scab begins to form the burn should be kept as dry as possible.

*Hypericum:* For deeper burns and scalds, also for burns which are becoming infected due to mistreatment. Apply as directed.

*Urtica Urens:* For simple burns and scalds, dilute and use to bathe a minor burn which can then be left open to the atmosphere.

## OINTMENTS

Useful for soothing minor burns and scalds. Apply liberally over the affected area as soon as possible. Either cover with a light dressing or leave exposed to the atmosphere.

*Hypericum and Urtica:* Apply locally to the affected area.

## HOMŒOPATHY

*Cantharis 30:* One or two doses a day for two to three days. Burns and scalds with stinging, smarting pains where blistering is predominant.

*Causticum 30:* One or two doses a day for two to three days. Severe and painful burns.

*Kali Bich 200:* Two doses twelve hours apart for severe pains in deep burns and old burn scarring.

*Urtica Urens 6 or 30:* Two or three doses over two to three days for simple, non-severe burns and scalds.

## AROMATHERAPY

*Lavender:* Used undiluted will soothe a burn, prevent infection, and help promote new tissue growth. The fragrance will also be useful for the trembling or panic that may accompany the burn. Apply liberally onto the affected area.

# C

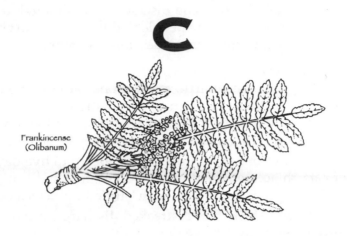

Frankincense
(Olibanum)

## CATARRH

Inflammation of the sensitive mucous membrane lining of nasal passages, throat and sinuses leads to an increased production of mucus, which in the healthy state is secreted to moisten and protect the area.

This may become a chronic problem, recurring each winter, in which case professional advice should be sought. There is a hereditary factor. For catarrh and congestion following a cold the suggested remedies below may be tried.

Diet is an important consideration; milk and all dairy products should be eliminated from the diet. Plenty of salads, vegetables, fresh fruits, garlic and onions need to be included.

(See also: SINUSITIS.)

### HERBS

*Bayberry, Elderflower, Eyebright, Golden Rod, Plantain:* These are anti-catarrhal and will bring relief. Combine and take as an infusion or tinctures three times a day for two to three weeks.

*Echinacea:* This may be added if infection is involved.

*Golden Seal:* This may be added to the mixture but

should be used with some discretion, for although it is extremely effective, some people find that it has a drying effect on the mucous membranes if use is prolonged.

## HOMŒOPATHY

In cases of chronic catarrh, professional advice should be sought, as there is often a miasmatic (inherited or acquired through suppression) background to this problem. For short-term relief the following may be helpful:

*Bryonia 6:* Take one three times a day for up to five days, for catarrh accompanied by offensive smell and coughing up of mucus. Headache with 'stuffed up' sensation.

*Calc Sulph 6X:* Thick, blood-streaked discharge of mucus. Three times a day for five days.

*Calc Sulph, Kali Sulph, Nat Sulph 6X:* For blocked sinuses and stuffed up sensation at the end of a cold. One three times a day for up to ten days.

*Hepar Sulph 6:* Thick yellow mucus with painful inflammation at the root of the nose. Worse in cold, dry wind. One three times a day for up to five days.

*Kali Bich 6:* Tough stringy plugs of mucus. Pain in the sinuses and at the root of the nose. Take one three times a day, for up to five days.

*Kali Mur 6X:* Thick, white, bland catarrh; stuffed up sensation of nose and ears. Three times a day for five to ten days.

*Kali Sulph 6X:* Yellow, slimy discharge of mucus from the nose; symptoms worse in the evenings and in warm rooms; longing for fresh air. Three times daily for five to ten days.

*Nat Mur 6X:* Watery discharge from nose and watering eyes. Sense of smell lost, much sneezing. One three times a day for up to ten days.

*Silica 6X:* Yellow-green nasal discharge with tendency to nose bleeds. Dry hard crusts in nose. Take one three times a day, for up to ten days.

AROMATHERAPY

*Eucalyptus, Frankincense (Olibanum), Pine, Ravensara:* Add two to three drops of the essential oils to a steam inhalation, or to a vegetable oil base, e.g. almond oil and rub onto the chest.

# CELLULITE

Cellulite is formed when the fat cells become interspersed with water and skin feels uneven and bumpy. Cellulite usually appears on the thighs, buttocks, and hips although it may appear virtually anywhere on the body.

Cellulite seems to be hormonally related and thus mild forms of it occur during different times of the menstrual cycle, or at times of hormonal upheaval such as pregnancy or the menopause. Use of the birth control pill might aggravate it. Bad circulation may also be a cause, therefore taking exercise and giving up smoking will help. In order to increase the circulation, try massaging with a body brush or a loofah.

Certain foods provoke fluid retention, and aggravate the cellulite problem, so treatment should include the avoidance of smoked or salty foods, sugar and refined carbohydrates.

HERBS

*Gotu Kola:* This herb has been proven during trials to help reduce cellulite. Make an infusion or use the tincture and take three times a day. Do not take it for more than six weeks in any one year.

*Birch, Cleavers, Dandelion Leaf, Fennel, Red Clover, Yellow Dock:* These herbs will gently cleanse the lymphatic system, have a mildly diuretic effect and rebalance the hormones. They may be taken in addition to *Gotu Kola.* Combine the herbs, make an infusion, or use the tinctures and drink three times daily for six weeks.

## HOMŒOPATHY

In order to get to the root of the problem, constitutional treatment will be necessary. The following tissue salts may be of help.

*Nat Phos 6X:* Regulates the distribution of intercellular fluids, most useful when acid conditions, e.g. rheumatism, digestive upsets or liver problems are found in association with cellulite. One twice daily for ten days.

*Nat Sulph 6X:* The excess water eliminator. Also helps clear out toxic fluids. Liverish symptoms may be present. One twice daily for ten days.

## AROMATHERAPY

*Black Pepper, Cypress, Fennel, Juniper, Lemon:* These help to eliminate toxins and disperse water. Add a few drops of each to a vegetable oil base, massage in morning and night, and also after a bath or sauna.

# CHICKENPOX (VARICELLA)

Chickenpox is one of the most contagious of all the childhood illnesses. The contagious period is from 24 hours before the rash starts to the time they scab over. Chickenpox may begin with a temperature, but often a rash is the first sign; this will appear in different parts of the body and will be extremely itchy. At first the spots are like dark red pimples; within a couple of hours they will have developed a small blister on top which resembles a drop of water, this will eventually form a scab and drop off.

Chickenpox is nearly always a mild disease, the most frequent complication being infection of the rash through scratching. As with all self-limiting childhood diseases it is important not to suppress the symptoms no matter what. Acute illness should be seen as an opportunity for the vitality to assert itself and throw off inherited or acquired toxicity.

## HERBS

INTERNAL

*Balm, Catnip, Chamomile, Elderflower, Heartsease:* Combine and drink an infusion three times daily, to soothe the patient and encourage rapid recovery.

EXTERNAL

*Chickweed, Lavender, Marigold, St John's Wort:* These may be combined to make a soothing and healing lotion, infuse, cool, and apply regularly with cotton wool. Sponge the body with diluted *Witchazel* to cool and relieve irritation if needed.

*Comfrey Oil or Ointment:* This may be massaged in once the pustules have stopped forming and the scabs have fallen off, to prevent scarring and promote skin healing.

*Stellaria Ointment:* Soothing and cooling for the rash. Apply locally.

## HOMŒOPATHY

*Ant Crud 30:* For a child who is irritable and does not want to be touched. Fearful itching worse when warm in bed. Two doses a day for two or three days.

*Ars Alb 30:* Large pus-filled eruptions, which may become open sores, burning pains accompany extreme chilliness. The patient is very restless and anxious. Two doses a day for two or three days.

*Belladonna 30:* For symptoms of fever, and red itching skin. Two doses a day for two or three days.

*Pulsatilla 6 or 30:* For a child who becomes clingy or weepy, and who is not thirsty despite fever. Take three doses of the 6th potency a day for five days, or one dose of the 30th potency a day for three days.

*Rhus Tox 6 or 30:* Eruptions which burn and itch, restlessness during the night. Take three doses of the 6th potency a day for five days, or one dose of the 30th potency a day for three days. This is the main remedy to ease discomfort and itching.

*Variolinum 30:* For a stubborn case of chickenpox, that is not responding well to treatment, or is dragging on too long. Give only two doses twelve hours apart.

AROMATHERAPY

*Roman Chamomile, Lavender, Tea Tree:* Add a few drops of each to a vegetable base oil and rub into the body for a soothing and healing effect.

# CHILBLAINS

These occur due to an inadequate supply of blood to the extremeties, i.e. fingers and toes, causing swelling, itching and burning sensations. A combination of treatment will be necessary to eradicate and prevent chilblains as several factors are involved. Locally, extremes of temperature should be avoided, well-fitting shoes should be worn with natural fibres next to the skin, applications to ease itching and soreness may be used. To assist circulation, constitutional treatment by a holistic practitioner is recommended. Diet is an important factor; salty foods and animal fats should be avoided. Foods rich in rutin, e.g. buckwheat, or bioflavonoid tablets will help strengthen the blood vessels and improve the circulation.

HERBS

INTERNAL

*Ginkgo, Ginger, Hawthorn, Prickly Ash:* Combined with a pinch of *Cayenne*, these will stimulate the circulation. Make an infusion and drink a cupful, or take as tinctures, three times daily for six weeks.

EXTERNAL

*Marigold, Myrrh, Witchazel Tinctures:* These should be combined and applied several times daily to unbroken chilblains, this will help reduce inflammation and heal the skin.

*Hypericum, Calendula Tinctures or Ointment:* Will promote healing of broken chilblains. Apply locally.

*Comfrey Ointment:* Will improve the quality of the skin in the area and help to reduce inflammation.

HOMŒOPATHY
Constitutional treatment is required to improve the circulation, and the following remedies may offer some specific relief.

*Agaricus 6:* Is indicated for burning and itching which is aggravated by the cold. Take one twice daily for ten days.

*Calc fluor 6X:* Improves the elasticity of the blood vessel walls and helps improve the circulation, it is indicated where cracks appear on the surface of the chilblains. One morning and night for ten days.

*Ferr Phos 6X:* For inflammation and to prevent infection. Three times a day when redness, heat and swelling is present.

*Pulsatilla 6:* For itching and burning which is worse for warmth. One twice daily for ten days.

AROMATHERAPY
*Chamomile, Cypress, Ginger, Lavender:* These will reduce inflammation, soothe the pain and itching, promoting cell regeneration. Add a few drops to a vegetable base oil, massage in morning and night, or use a few drops in a foot bath.

# CIRCULATION

Circulation is the constant flow of blood and other body fluids in the organism. If there is an imbalance in this flow it can lead to many disorders; including cramp, angina pectoris, high blood pressure, low blood pressure, thrombosis and varicose veins. Poor circulation is particularly associated with heart problems, degeneration of the blood vessels and increased blood viscosity. It is most notably true of circulatory disease that prevention is better than trying to cure a worn out body that is manifesting symptoms. To prevent any circulatory diseases, lifestyle should be considered.

Diet is crucial; there should be a low intake of animal fats, meat, butter, oils, cakes and dairy products. Salt should be avoided, and increase foods rich in vitamin C. Regular, although not necessarily strenuous, exercise is important to tone the circulation. It is also advisable to stop smoking and keep the intake of alcohol to a moderate amount.

There is a close correlation between the levels of stress in life, and problems occurring in the cardio-vascular system. Therefore it is necessary to deal with the underlying causes of stress and tension as well as its physical manifestation. There are many forms of relaxation and emotional integration therapies available at the present time and these may be of great benefit when trying to improve physical and psychological health. Sudden changes in previously established circulation patterns should be assessed by a physician. Acupuncture is particularly recommended for this complaint.

## HERBS

*Dandelion Leaves, Motherwort:* If the heart is weak and fails to circulate blood efficiently through the kidneys, or when the blood vessels are weak; a build up of water in certain areas of the body may occur. Combine and drink three times a day for one month.

*Hawthorn Berries, Hawthorn Tops:* These make a useful heart tonic, drink an infusion or take the tinctures three times daily for six weeks.

*Ginkgo:* This is a useful circulatory tonic, and may be added to the above mixture, especially when the peripheral circulation is in need of stimulation.

## HOMŒOPATHY

Again most benefit will be gained by constitutional treatment from a practitioner. In cases where support for another therapy is required, the following remedies may prove useful:

*Calc Fluor 6X:* Will strengthen and give elasticity to the blood vessel walls. Take one three times daily for two weeks.

*Calc Phos 6X:* For those who are generally run down, with slow and weak circulation. Two a day for two weeks.

*Kali Mur 6X:* For sluggish circulation and tendency of blood to clot too quickly. One twice daily for two weeks.

AROMATHERAPY

*Lavender, Marjoram, Ylang Ylang:* Useful oils for reducing high blood pressure, being soothing and calming. They will help to relieve tension and promote relaxation.

*Cypress, Ginger, Grapefruit:* These are good general circulation tonics. Add two to three drops of the essential oils to a warm bath or dilute in a vegetable oil base and massage into the skin.


## COLDS

Colds are an attempt by the body to express disharmony. They are an opportunity for the system to discharge unwanted waste matter. They may also be an indication that the person needs to slow down and rest, or to look at some unexpressed emotional difficulties; colds after all share many of the symptoms of grief, e.g. weeping. Thus the aim of treatment should not be to suppress the indicator (and stay out of balance), but to gently restore health and harmony.

Because many of the symptoms of a cold are due to increased mucus secretion, attention to diet is advisable. In particular eliminating all dairy products, wheat products, and concentrated orange juice. It will also help to increase intake of foods that are natural sources of vitamin C, i.e. fresh fruit and vegetables.

HERBS

*Elderflower, Peppermint, Yarrow:* A traditional mixture to relieve the symptoms of feverish colds. Make an infusion and drink a cupful three times a day. If feverishness is marked, add *Boneset*. Add *Red Sage* if there is throat inflammation. Hot *Lemon* and *Honey* is also recommended. Freshly grated *Ginger* may be added to any of the above infusions for a warming effect.

## HOMŒOPATHY

*ABC 6 or 30 (Aconite, Belladonna, Chamomilla):* A combination remedy. For the beginning of colds and feverish types of illnesses. Will keep you going during the first stages of a cold, and may prevent it from dragging on too long. Especially suitable for children. Take three times a day for two to three days.

*Aconite 30:* Sudden onset of cold symptoms, after exposure to cold or cold winds. Sore throat, headache and restlessness may be present. One three times a day for the first day or two.

*Allium Cepa 30:* Common cold symptoms with much sneezing, watering eyes and acrid nasal discharge. One three times a day for two to three days.

*Belladonna 30:* Feels feverish and congested. Sore throat and cough may be present. One three times a day for two or three days.

*Bryonia 30:* Colds descending to the chest. 'Heavy' headache. One three times a day for two or three days.

*Gelsemium 30:* Hot and cold shivering. Aching muscles. Colds that develop into flu like symptoms. One three times a day for two or three days.

*Kali Mur 6X:* If there is white mucous and general congested feeling. One three times a day for three to four days.

*Nat Mur 6X:* Watery nasal discharge, also eyes may water. Loss of taste and smell. One three times a day for three to four days.

## AROMATHERAPY

*Eucalyptus, Lemon, Pine, Ravensara, Tea Tree:* Choose one or two from these essential oils, add to a vegetable base oil, and massage onto the chest. A few drops may be put onto a handkerchief or pillow, or alternatively added to hot water as a steam inhalation.

*Ginger:* Add ten drops to a basin of warm water for a foot-bath.

## COLD SORES

Many people suffer from this virus, which does not manifest itself until the resistance of the body is lowered, and results in blisters forming around the mouth, or occasionally nose and eyes. The blisters start as reddish lumps and develop into watery vesicles before a scab forms. Constitutional treatment is recommended to deal with the underlying cause, although the following may relieve the occasional sore.

### HERBS

#### INTERNAL

*Balm:* This herb is proven to be active against the herpes simplex virus when used externally. Dab on the cooled infusion three times a day or use the tincture to shorten the duration of the symptoms.

*Echinacea, Yarrow:* These immune-system stimulating herbs may be added to *Balm* for stubborn cases.

#### EXTERNAL

*Golden Seal, Myrrh Tincture:* These dabbed on the sores will speed healing.

*Marigold and St John's Wort Infusion or Tincture:* These are soothing and healing. Dab on to affected area.

*Comfrey Ointment:* This will help the skin after the scabs have gone.

### HOMŒOPATHY

*Ars Alb 30:* Sores are accompanied by a burning sensation, and sense of irritability. One twice daily for three to five days.

*Hepar Sulph 30:* Sores with pus formation, acutely sensitive to touch and cold. One twice daily for three to five days.

*Nat Mur 30:* Herpes blisters containing clear liquid, lips may be cracked, sores often appear during a cold. Take one two times daily for three to four days.

*Rhus Tox 30:* Inflamed blisters filled with yellowish, watery fluid; associated with burning and itching. One twice daily for three to five days.

AROMATHERAPY
*Niaouli, Tea Tree:* Apply undiluted to the affected area.

## COLIC

Colic is generally experienced as a spasmodic pain in the abdomen. In a baby it is usually a digestive upset causing the baby to cry in pain and pass wind. Most infants outgrow it in three to four months, but this can be distressing at the time. In older children and adults a warm hot water bottle hugged to the stomach often gives relief. One should consult a practitioner if it is a recurring symptom, or if there is any doubt about the diagnosis.

HERBS
*Caraway, Fennel, Ginger, Wild Yam:* Make an infusion and drink as often as necessary.

*Caraway, Dill Seeds:* For babies these can help to relieve the gripe pains. Use one teaspoon, for one third of a pint. Infuse and give to the baby in a bottle or by teaspoon after feeding.

*Chamomile:* A soothing tea useful for babies and young children. Make an infusion to drink when required.

HOMŒOPATHY
*Chamomilla 30:* Resdess and irritable, due to a pain in the stomach, and may be accompanied by diarrhoea. Take one three times a day or as necessary. Useful for young children.

*Colocynth30:* Violent griping pains in stomach and abdomen. Patient bends double to alleviate the pain. Flatulent colic. Repeat as required.

*Mag Phos 6X:* Helps colic that is better from warmth and gently rubbing the abdomen. Cramping, spasmodic pains. One every few hours as necessary.

AROMATHERAPY

*Chamomile, Orange, Peppermint, Yarrow:* Blend a few drops of one or two with almond oil and gently massage into the stomach.

## COLITIS

Colitis is an inflammation of part of the colon or large intestine. It is an increasingly common disturbance of our modern high-stress lifestyle. If the problem is longstanding or with a hereditary background, only persistent careful treatment by a qualified therapist will be of lasting benefit. This condition will respond to a change of diet; based upon non-acidic, non-irritant foods. Avoid dairy products, bran products, pulses, rich fatty foods, and stimulants such as tea, coffee and alcohol.

Symptoms are marked by colicky pains after eating, with constipation or diarrhoea and depression. Check with a doctor for an accurate diagnosis for these symptoms are shared by other illnesses. Colitis can respond quickly to alternative methods of treatment.

Acupuncture has been found to be of much benefit. Also any sufferer of colitis could investigate the Bach flower remedies to assist in bringing about change in the stress patterns and mental habits which lie in the background of this problem.

HERBS

The following herbs may bring relief and ease discomfort.

*Comfrey, Marigold, Marshmallow Root, Meadowsweet, Peppermint:* Infuse and drink three times a day for up to six weeks.

*Fenugreek:* Contains healing mucilage. Make a decoction of the crushed seeds and take three times daily. May be taken in conjunction with the above blend of herbs.

*Slippery Elm:* Soothes and heals the colon. A teaspoon dissolved in warm water taken three times a day.

HOMŒOPATHY
Constitutional treatment with a qualified practitioner is recommended for this condition.

AROMATHERAPY
A relaxing massage and advice from an experienced aromatherapist will be of benefit.

## CONCUSSION

A fall or blow to the head resulting in confusion or temporary loss of consciousness; this may cause a severe disturbance in the body and symptoms can be delayed for several hours. This condition is serious and experienced medical help is required immediately.

*Arnica 30 or 200,* or *Five Flower Remedy* may be helpful to administer whilst help is being sought.

## CONJUNCTIVITIS

An inflammation and swelling of the conjunctiva of the eye. The affected eye will water and look bloodshot. When infected by cold viruses the discharge is clear and watery; bacterial infections result in thick, yellow-green discharges; allergic conjunctivitis is accompanied by itching.

When the discharge dries during sleep the eyelids may stick together.

When treating the eyes take care to wash utensils and hands carefully, and use cool, boiled or distilled water only to apply to the area.

If symptoms persist beyond three days, or if they are associated with any loss of vision, or pain in the eye, or following an injury or possible exposure to flying fragments of metal or grit, then seek urgent medical advice.

(See also: EYE INJURIES, EYE STRAIN.)

## HERBS

### INTERNAL

*Cleavers, Echinacea, Eyebright, Golden Seal:* Use a combination of these herbs to fight the infection and soothe the eyes. Make a decoction by simmering a teaspoon of the mixed herbs to a mug of water for ten minutes. Strain and drink a cupful three times a day for up to two weeks.

### EXTERNAL

*Eyebright, Golden Seal (half), Marigold:* Use these herbs singly or in combination. Make an infusion using a heaped teaspoon of herb to a teacup of boiling water and stand until cool. Strain and use the solution to bathe the eye. Or use one to two drops of tincture in a little cool, boiled water.

## HOMŒOPATHY

*Apis 30:* Swelling and puffiness of the eyelids. Stinging and burning pains in the eye worse in a warm room. Redness. One dose three times a day for three days.

*Belladonna 30:* Throbbing sensation. Redness, inflammation and hot, watery, discharge. One dose three times a day for three days.

*Euphrasia 30:* Acrid tears, thick discharge, sensation of sand in the eye. One dose three times a day for three days.

*Pulsatilla 30:* Thick, yellow-green discharge. Itching and burning sensation. Often following a cold. Symptoms better in the fresh air. One dose three times a day for three days.

### EXTERNAL

*Euphrasia Tincture:* Add three of four drops of the tincture to a little cool, boiled water and bathe the affected eye.

## CONSTIPATION

There is much controversy as to how often it is 'healthy' or 'normal' to pass a stool. Generally speaking if bowel movements are less frequent than every two days, or straining is required, and stomach pains are evident, then constipation is present to some extent.

We get many people in the shop requiring laxatives. These are unadvisable as they can be habit forming, and inhibit the bowels' normal functioning. There are two main forms of laxative: one irritates the walls of the colon causing expulsion of waste matter, the other absorbs moisture from the intestinal lining thereby increasing fluids in the forming stools.

Constipation can be helped by a change of diet, increasing fluid intake, fresh fruit and vegetables. Exercise is of great help, and it will also be useful to look at any underlying emotional tensions or stress.

An ongoing change in a previously established pattern of bowel habit should be assessed by a physician.

### HERBS

*Cascara Sagrada, Fennel, Liquorice, Marshmallow Root, Rhubarb Root, Senna Leaves:* Make an infusion and drink one cup a day, in the evening. This will alleviate the odd bout of constipation. Anything more persistent should be referred to an herbalist.

*Psyllium Seeds (Isphagula):* A gentle bulk laxative. Add one to two teaspoonfuls to water and take twice daily for several days.

### HOMŒOPATHY

If this complaint is chronic, seek advice from a trained practitioner. For acute cases the following may be of help.

*Alumina 6 or 30:* Inactivity of the colon, with soft stool; constipation common to travellers. Take three doses of the 6th potency a day for five days, or one dose of the 30th potency a day for three days.

*Nat Mur 6:* Constipation when caused from lack of moisture in the intestines. Hard, dry, black, lumpy stools difficult to pass, accompanied by dull, heavy headache. Take one three times a day for three days.

*Nux Vom 30:* Urging for stool that does not come. A small stool may be passed, with the feeling some is left behind. One or two doses.

*Sepia 30:* Ineffectual urging, sensation of lump in the rectum, not relieved by passing a stool. Feeling of heaviness and sluggishness. Constipation of pregnancy. One or two doses.

## AROMATHERAPY
There are many essential oils to help tone, detoxify and relax the body. Massage would be of great benefit to relieve tension and a visit to an aromatherapist is recommended.

*Black Pepper, Fennel, Grapefruit, Rosemary:* In an acute situation, these oils diluted in a massage base oil and rubbed on the abdomen may help.

## BACH FLOWER REMEDIES
These could be very useful to change habits, and help underlying emotional or stress patterns. See the list in the Appendix or consult a practitioner.

# CONVALESCENCE
After a debilitating illness or a long winter when the body's natural defences have been weakened and one is prone to illness and infections, the following may be of help. (See also: APPETITE LOSS.)

## HERBS
*Alfalfa, Balm, Nettle, Vervain:* These will soothe and gently tonify the system. Combine and make an infusion to drink three times a day.

*Siberian Ginseng:* An excellent tonic to aid recovery from illness. Take the tincture three times a day for several weeks.

## HOMŒOPATHY

*Calc Phos 6X:* Is of great help as it tones up the system and aids the assimilation processes. Take three times a day for two weeks.

*Phos Ac 30:* For exhaustion and apathy, following trauma or illness. Take only two doses eight hours apart.

## AROMATHERAPY

*Geranium, Lavender, Melissa, Rosemary:* Choose one or two of these oils and add a couple of drops to a warm bath, or apply diluted in a massage base.

# CORNS

These are often formed by pressure from ill-fitting shoes, and poor posture, creating a hard layer of dead tissue, which can be quite painful. It is advisable to visit a chiropodist if the corns are at all severe.

Soak the foot in very hot water until the skin becomes soft, and gently peel away dead tissue.

## HERBS

*Calendula Tincture, Hypericum:* These added to the water promote healing and prevent infection.

*Comfrey, Marshmallon, Slippery Elm, Garlic:* Infused and applied as a compress may be of help.

*Lemon Juice:* Also softens the skin.

## HOMŒOPATHY

*Calc Fluor 6X:* For hard, calloused skin. Take twice daily for ten days.

*Ferr Phos 6X:* For acute inflammatory pain. One three times a day.

## AROMATHERAPY

*Chamomile, Lavender, Lemon:* Combine and add a few drops to a warm foot bath. This combination of oils may also be diluted in a vegetable base oil and massaged into the foot.

*Tea Tree:* Apply undiluted and massage into the corn to relieve pain and prevent infection.

## COUGHS

Coughing is a reflex action as an attempt to expel foreign matter from the air passages. Mucus is produced as a response to dust, bacterial infection and other irritants. Arresting a cough by use of cough suppressants is therefore undesirable, and can cause a deeper infection. Avoid dairy products and other mucus-forming foods.

A simple and soothing cough remedy suitable for adults and children can be made from a slice of fresh lemon, a teaspoon of honey, and a few drops of *Elderberry* tincture added to hot water. (See also: ASTHMA, BRONCHITIS, WHOOPING COUGH.)

## CRAMP

This is a painful spasm of muscles which may be due to circulatory problems. Consult a practitioner if the cramping occurs frequently.

(See also: COLIC, MENSTRUAL PROBLEMS.)

### HERBS

*Balm, Cramp Bark:* These herbs as an infusion may help to alleviate the problem. Drink a cupful as required.

### HOMŒOPATHY

*Arnica 30:* Cramp after over-exertion of muscles; system feels sore and bruised. One dose as necessary.

*Cuprum 30:* Severe cramping of the extremities, worse at night. One dose as required.

*Mag Phos 6X:* For muscular, stomach and menstrual cramps. Alleviated by rubbing and warmth. Dosage as required.

AROMATHERAPY
*Aniseed, Basil, Marjoram:* Add two drops of each to a little base massage oil, and rub into the area.

# CROUP

A harsh cough accompanied by rapid, loud breathing; occurs mostly in children at night. Emergency care is needed if symptoms have no relief after twenty minutes, or whenever the child has severe breathing difficulties. Be cautious: this is a potentially serious condition. A traditional remedy is to provide a steamy atmosphere by boiling a kettle in the room.

HERBS
*Eucalyptus:* This may be used as an inhalation. Put some of the leaves in a basin, pour on boiling water, and stand it in the patient's room.

*Catnip, Chamomile, Coltsfoot:* A soothing tea that will also relieve spasms. Make an infusion and drink a cupful as required.

HOMŒOPATHY
*Aconite 30:* At onset, if there is a lot of fear and worse at night. One or two doses as required.

*Hepar Sulph 30 or Spongia 30:* If *Aconite* brings no relief. Child wakes feeling suffocated, with loud violent cough and loss of voice. *Spongia* if worse before midnight and *Hepar Sulph* afterwards. One or two doses as required.

AROMATHERAPY
*Cypress, Eucalyptus:* These two oils could be diluted and sprayed in the room, or placed in a bowl of hot water near the child to inhale the steam.

*Lavender:* Can be used as a compress to soothe the child, apply on the head or chest.

BACH FLOWER REMEDIES
*Five Flower Remedy:* This may help a fearful child.

## CYSTITIS

A urinary tract infection which can be most uncomfortable. The symptoms are an urgent need to urinate, frequency of urination, accompanied by burning sensation. If there is fever, lower back pain, blood or sediment in the urine, we advise you to seek urgent medical attention, as the kidneys may be infected, leading to chronic damage.

Professional help should be sought if the condition is recurrent. The following remedies may help a mild, acute attack.

### HERBS

*Buchu, Cornsilk, Couchgrass, Marshmallow Leaves:* Combine, infuse and drink a cupful every two hours.

### HOMŒOPATHY

*Apis 30:* Frequent urge to urinate, last few drops sting. Two or three doses.

*Cantharis 30:* Persistent and violent urge to urinate, with burning, cutting or stabbing pains. Two or three doses.

*Merc Cor 30:* Urine is a dark colour, burning sensation. Worse at night. Two or three doses for three days.

*Nux Vom 30:* Cutting, burning pains; feels chilly and irritable. Worse at night. Two or three doses a day for three days.

### AROMATHERAPY

*Bergamot, Cedarwood, Cypress, Juniper, Lavender, Sandalwood:* Combine one or two drops of two or three of the oils in a little massage base oil and apply to the abdomen, or add to a warm bath.

# D

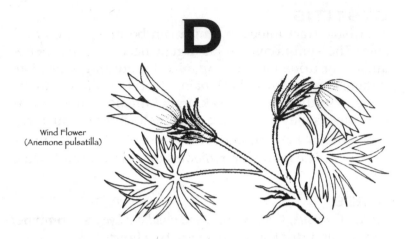

Wind Flower
(Anemone pulsatilla)

## DANDRUFF

Dandruff seems to be an indication of your general state of health. It is in fact dead cells flaking from the scalp. Strong detergents as in anti-dandruff shampoos should be avoided as they are only a short-term solution and may cause scalp irritation if used frequently. Mild shampoos such as *Nettle* are recommended. Best results will come from a visit to a qualified practitioner especially when dandruff is severe.

HERBS

EXTERNAL
*Nettles:* Make an infusion and massage into scalp daily.

INTERNAL
*Burdock, Heartsease:* Mix and make an infusion using one
teaspoon per cup. Drink three cups a day.

HOMŒOPATHY
Homœopathic tissue salts may be helpful.
*Kali Mur 6X:* Copious white dandruff. One dose morning
and night for ten days.

*Kali Sulph 6X:* Poor conditions of scalp with flaking and scaling. Yellow dandruff. One dose morning and night for ten days.

AROMATHERAPY

*Cedarwood, Lavender, Rosemary:* Add ten drops of each to a suitable vegetable base oil, e.g. coconut oil. Massage into scalp, leave on overnight before washing off. Will help improve the condition of hair and scalp.

## DENTAL PROBLEMS
(See also: ABSCESS, GINGIVITIS, TEETHING, TOOTHACHE.)

HOMŒOPATHY

*Arnica 30:* This remedy can considerably lessen the physical trauma and aid recovery following a visit to the dentist. Take one dose one hour before treatment and one dose one hour afterwards.

BACH FLOWER REMEDIES

*Mimulus:* For anticipatory fear. Take a couple of drops in a little water as often as required before visiting the dentist.

## DEPRESSION
There are many interpretations of what depression means. We recognise that there are times when states of feeling low and unhappy with yourself and the world hit you unsuspectingly. Sometimes events such as the loss of a loved one can trigger depression.

Some physical reasons can provoke this state: such as after giving birth, after illness, after an operation or as a result of taking drugs, etc. We will list some helpful remedies to take when there is an obvious cause, or when the depression is of a non-severe nature; but basically we feel that much depression springs from an attitude that is common in our society in which we tend to lose touch with our purpose for existence and our inner sense of creativity. We will use difficult circumstances and various incidents as the excuse, but really we feel that depression is the outcome of lack of communication of initial emotional reactions. Failure or inability to recognise and express these primary emotions leads to suppression; this develops into a complication and confusion of emotions, which may progress into feelings of depression and a loss of our sense of worth. This is why lifting depression is often a process, made up of a number of steps, rather than a single solution.

Some symptoms of depression are: loss of appetite, sleeplessness, anxiety, lassitude and lack of sexual interest.

The use of anti-depressants we feel is counter productive. There are nowadays many forms of group or individual therapy which may be of help. Some assessment should be made (by a qualified practitioner) of the severity of the depression: in particular regarding the presence of suicidal ideas. Milder forms of depression will usually respond to a combination of positive lifestyle changes in conjunction with natural remedies such as suggested below. Regular exercise and regular meditation can be very helpful.

HERBS

*St John's Wort:* This has been proven in clinical trials to be effective at relieving mild to moderate depression. It is also specific for SAD or 'winter blues' and menopausal depression or anxiety. *St John's Wort* may interact with certain forms of medication so check with a practitioner if you need to take prescription drugs.

*Balm, Scullcap, Vervain:* These herbs are useful and soothing nervines, that will act to lift the spirits. Mix the herbs and make an infusion using one heaped teaspoonful of herbs to a cupful of boiling water, or use the tinctures. This may be taken three times a day as required or for up to four weeks.

*Damiana:* Add this to the above mixture if there is weakness and debility associated with the depression.

Best results will be obtained from a visit to a qualified herbalist.

## HOMŒOPATHY
We feel that when dealing with depression, any homœopathic remedy should be prescribed by a qualified homœopath, as it is constitutional treatment that will be of lasting benefit.

## AROMATHERAPY
A course of treatment by a qualified aromatherapist could be of great value in cases of depression.

*Basil, Clary Sage, Jasmine, Neroli, Rose:* These oils have an uplifting effect. Add a few drops of the one of your choice to an essential oil burner and fragrance the room, blend in a massage oil, or add to a base oil and use in the bath.

## BACH FLOWER REMEDIES
Bach flower remedies can be of great benefit in the treatment of depression. We suggest that you spend some time going through the relevant literature, starting with the list in the Appendix, and choosing the appropriate remedies for yourself. Alternatively, one may visit a practitioner for guidance about the most useful remedies to take.


# DIARRHOEA
There are many causes of diarrhoea. Chronic (long-term) diarrhoea as experienced for example in colitis or diverticulitis should be referred to a qualified practitioner. Unfamiliar or spoilt foods can cause an inflammation or irritation of the stomach lining or intestinal tract; diarrhoea will result as an attempt to eliminate them. Emotional circumstances such as grief, exam tension etc. or travelling may also cause diarrhoea. If the diarrhoea is severe, or if it continues for more than twenty-four hours,

consult a medical practitioner because diarrhoea can be an indication of something more serious. It is extremely important to alert a medical practitioner about any case of diarrhoea occurring in babies and young children, as dehydration can set in quickly, and this is a very dangerous situation: if in doubt this is a time when it is vital to err on the side of caution.

General care includes drinking plenty of water and eating only plain foods until the digestive system has had a chance to settle down.

HERBS

*Chamomile, Marshmallow, Meadowsweet:* Combine the above herbs and make an infusion using one heaped teaspoon of herbs to a cupful of boiling water. Drink a cupful every few hours to soothe irritation and counteract any acidity.

*Agrimony:* Add this to the above mixture for childhood diarrhoea.

*Ginger, Peppermint:* Add these to any of the above if griping pains are present.

*Slippery Elm:* Stir a heaped teaspoonful of *Slippery Elm* powder into a cup of warm water. Drink a cupful three times a day. This will soothe the digestive system and provide some nourishment.

HOMŒOPATHY

There are many homœopathic remedies for diarrhoea and if you are registered with a homœopathic practitioner it is best to consult them for advice, this is a must when dealing with young children. The following remedies are some of those most commonly found to be of assistance in treating diarrhoea. For best results it may be necessary to try two or three different remedies as the symptoms change.

*Ars Alb 30:* Watery, burning diarrhoea. Results of bad food or excessive eating of fruit. The patient is restless, anxious and chilly, and desires sips of water. One dose every few hours as required.

*Bryonia 30:* Gushing diarrhoea worse whenever the patient moves. Dry parched lips and great thirst. Take two or three doses spread throughout the day.

*Chamomilla 6 or 30:* Diarrhoea in children. Colicky pains, green or watery stool. The child is whiney and irritable.

*Colocynth 30:* Diarrhoea resulting from food poisoning with cramping, colicky pains. The pains are better for pressure and bending double. One dose every few hours as required.

*Mag Phos 30:* Cramping pains accompanying diarrhoea. The patient is chilly. One dose every few hours as required.

*Merc Sol 30:* Offensive, smelly, watery, bloody or mucousy stools. Constant urging and straining to pass a stool. Diarrhoea worse at night. Two or three doses spread over one or two days.

*Nat Phos 30:* Sour-smelling, acidic stools. Summer diarrhoea from eating too much fruit. One dose every few hours as required.

*Podophyllum 30:* Gushing, watery stools passed painlessly. Gurgling in the abdomen. Diarrhoea worse after eating or drinking, and worse in hot weather. One dose every few hours as required.

*Pulsatilla 30:* Diarrhoea after rich food. Patient dislikes a stuffy room and is worse at night. Thirstless, depressed and weepy patient. One dose every few hours as required.

AROMATHERAPY

*Chamomile, Geranium, Sandalwood:* Add a few drops of any of these oils to a vegetable oil base and lightly massage onto the abdomen to soothe the digestive tract.

*Cinnamon, Thyme:* These oils may be used in a burner or sprayed in the room as a disinfectant.

# E

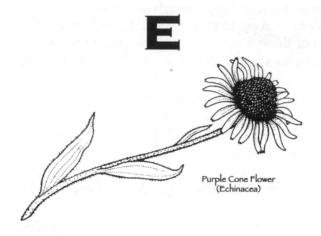

Purple Cone Flower
(Echinacea)

## EARACHE

Earache is particularly common in children, it is often a painful and distressing problem. Pain is caused by inflammation, or a build up of fluids causing pressure on the eardrum. Infection of the middle ear, which is indicated by redness and swelling in the outer ear, can be serious and we suggest you get medical attention as soon as possible. Any pain or swelling in the bony area behind or under the ear requires immediate medical attention as this may develop into inflammation of the brain which is an extremely dangerous condition. The presence of a discharge from the ear indicates a perforation of the ear drum. Care must be taken to prevent the entry of water, shampoo, etc., until the drum has fully healed.

Any residual hearing loss, after the acute episode is over, should be professionally assessed: this can easily go unnoticed in children. Recurrent earaches can result in permanent hearing loss so constitutional treatment by a qualified alternative therapist should be considered to prevent attacks recurring.

### HERBS

*Chamomile, Echinacea, Golden Rod, Golden Seal:* Combine the herbs and make a decoction using one teaspoon of herbs to a cupful of water and simmer for ten minutes. Drink a cupful three times a day to reduce inflammation and prevent infection. Children may not like this bitter mixture so it may be worth using herbal tinctures instead: combine the tinctures and dilute in a wine glass of warm water to drink three times a day.

*Mullein Oil:* Add a few drops slightly warmed to a piece of cotton wool and place gently inside the outer ear.

HOMŒOPATHY

*Aconite 6 or 30:* Sudden attack of earache after exposure to cold winds. One 6 potency every few hours for two to three days, or two doses of the 30 potency eight hours apart.

*Belladonna 6 or 30:* Throbbing pain in the ear. Ear looks red and feels hot. Pain accompanied with fever. Dosage as for *Aconite.*

*Chamomilla 6 or 30:* Earache in teething children. Child is whiney and intolerant, the pain feels unbearable to them. One cheek looks red. Dosage as for *Aconite.*

*Ferrum Phos 6X:* Helpful at the beginning stage of inflammation when there are few distinguishing features. Ear feels hot and looks red. One dose every three hours.

*Hepar Sulph 6 or 30:* Useful when pus has formed. Stitching pains in the ear. Pains are worse at night. Patient is feverish, irritable and sweaty. Dosage as for *Aconite.*

*Kali Mur 6X or 30:* Blocked up feeling in the ear; diminished hearing. This may be useful after the pain has subsided but hearing is impaired. One dose of 6X potency three times a day for five days or just two doses of 30 potency eight hours apart.

*Pulsatilla 6 or 30:* Pain as from pressure in the ear. Pains worse from warmth and at night. Child is weepy and craves attention. Thick yellow discharge. Dosage as for *Aconite..*

*Silica 6 or 30:* Pain and swelling in the area around the ear. Yellow or green discharge. Weak, tired and chilly patient. Dosage as for Aconite.

## AROMATHERAPY

*Lavender:* Put two or three drops on a piece of cotton wool and hold against the ear to soothe pain and reduce inflammation. Or dilute Lavender Oil in a massage base to gently massage in around the ear area.

# ECZEMA

Eczema is a name given to a wide variety of skin disorders. As it is a deep-rooted condition with a variety of causes, it should be treated constitutionally by a qualified practitioner. Herbalism, naturopathy, homœopathy and aromatherapy can all be very successful in dealing with this distressing problem. Symptoms include redness, itching, flaking and weeping skin. The use of strong chemical ointments, whilst effective in the short term, have serious long term side-effects and are not curative, merely suppressive.

The following suggestions may be used in conjunction with remedies prescribed by a qualified practitioner, but check with them first.

## HERBS

### INTERNAL

*Burdock, Chickweed, Cleavers, Heartsease, Marigold, Red Clover:* Combine the above herbs, make an infusion using one teaspoon of herbs to one teacupful of boiling water, and drink a cupful three times a day for up to six weeks.

*Echinacea, Wild Yam:* Add these to the mixture if your eczema is prone to getting infected.

### EXTERNAL

*Chickweed, Marigold:* Make an infusion using one tablespoon of herbs to one pint of boiling water. Leave to stand until cool, strain, then bathe the affected areas.

*Calendula Ointment:* A soothing and healing ointment that will help prevent infection.

*Stellaria Ointment:* This will help soothe any itching.

## HOMŒOPATHY
We recommend that you see a qualified homœopath to get the full benefit of homœopathic treatment.

## AROMATHERAPY
*Chamomile, Lavender, Yarrow*: Combine the oils. Use as a compress, in a warm bath, or dilute in a suitable vegetable massage oil to apply to the affected parts. Do a patch test on the inside of your wrist or elbow before using any new essential oil on sensitive skin.

# EYE INJURIES
Because the eyes are so delicate, any eye injury should be examined by a physician for possible complications. Loose foreign bodies in the eye should be flushed out with plenty of cool, clean water.
(See also: CONJUNCTIVITIS.)

## HERBS
*Witchazel*: Dilute distilled *Witchazel* in cool, boiled water. Dip some clean cotton wool in the solution and hold over the eye to soothe inflammation and bruising.

*Chamomile, Eyebright*: An infusion may be drunk to strengthen the eyes and reduce inflammation.

*Tinctures*

*Euphrasia*: Use to soothe irritation or inflammation. Add one to two drops of the tincture to a little cool, boiled water in an eyebath and gently bathe the eyes.

*Marigold*: Use after a foreign body has been expelled to soothe the eye and help prevent infection. Add one or two drops to a little cool, boiled water and use as an eyewash.

## HOMŒOPATHY
*Arnica 30*: Useful following any injury. Prevents haemorrhage, reduces bruising and helps with shock. Three times a day for two or three days.

*Ledum 30:* For a black eye with bruising and swelling. Take two or three doses over two days.

*Silica 30:* Will help to expel a foreign body from the eye. One dose three times a day for three days.

*Symphytum 6 or 30:* For injury to the eyeball. Two doses of 30 potency a day for three days, or three doses of 6 potency a day for five days.

## AROMATHERAPY

*Lavender:* Add one drop of essential oil to an eyebath with cool, boiled water in. Dip in a piece of cotton wool and hold over the affected eye taking care that none of the oil gets into the eye.

# EYE STRAIN

Cold teabags, placed on the eye are very effective.

## HERBS

*Cucumber:* A slice of cucumber placed over each eye is very cooling and soothing.

*Eyebright:* Make an infusion, cool, strain and bathe the eye. Or use one drop of the tincture in a little cool, boiled water. This tea can also be taken internally to strengthen the eyes.

## HOMŒOPATHY

*Ruta 6:* Eyes red, hot and painful from reading fine print, sewing, etc. Vision seems dim. One dose three times a day for five days.

## AROMATHERAPY

*Lavender:* Add one drop of essential oil to an eyebath with cool, boiled water in. Dip in a piece of cotton wool and hold over the affected eye taking care that none of the oil gets into the eye.

# F

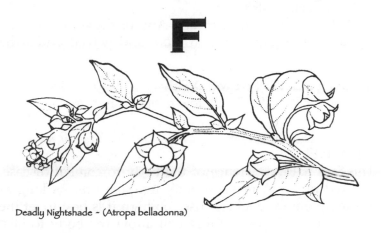

Deadly Nightshade ~ (Atropa belladonna)

## FAINTING

This is a reflex action as a result of temporary loss of oxygen to the brain; often resulting from intense fear, low blood pressure, lack of air, e.g., stuffy room, emotional upset, or intense pain. Basic first-aid can be given. Sit with head lower than body until one feels better. If fainting recurs, seek medical advice.

### HERBS

*Peppermint, Rosemary, St John's Wort:* Any of these can be used as a tea for occasional fainting. Make an infusion and drink a cupful every two to three hours.

### HOMŒOPATHY

*Chamomilla 30:* Fainting from severe pain. Use one or more doses as required.

*China 30:* Fainting due to loss of vital fluids. Use one or more dose as required.

*Coffea 30:* Fainting from excitement. Use one or more doses as required.

*Ignatia 30:* Fainting due to emotional shock or hysteria. Use one or more doses as required.

*Pulsatilla 30:* Fainting from hot, stuffy atmosphere. Use one or more doses as required.

## AROMATHERAPY
*Lavender, Peppermint, Rosemary:* Any of these can be used placed on a pad of cotton wool and waved under the nose.

## BACH FLOWER REMEDIES
*Five Flower Remedy:* Take a few drops as required.

# FEVER
This is a natural defence of the body to combat disease, marked by an increase in body temperature. As long as the temperature does not rise too high it is best to let the fever run its course, as this will allow the body to heal itself. For a mild fever the following remedies will assist; remembering plenty of fluids should be taken and chilliness prevented. Sponging the body with tepid water will help. If fever continues to rise, consult a physician.

It is especially important to keep a close watch on children, as they may develop convulsions during a high fever and emergency medical advice must be sought if there seems any likelihood of this occurring.

## HERBS
*Boneset, Echinacea, Elderflower, Yarrow:* Combine and drink an infusion three times a day to reduce fever and help fight off infection.

*Balm, Catnip, Chamomile:* This can also be drunk as a soothing tea throughout a fever. These herbs are also suitable for children.

## HOMŒOPATHY
*Aconite 30:* For sudden onset after exposure to cold wind. Anxious, fearful, dry skin and mouth. Take one dose of the 30th potency and repeat as necessary.

*Ars Alb 30:* Fluctuating temperature, restless, anxious, fearful, chilly patient. Thirsty for sips of water. One dose of the 30th potency twice a day for three days.

*Belladonna 30:* Restless, agitated, glassy eyes, red face, burning hot skin and delirium. Take one dose of the 30th potency and repeat as necessary.

*Ferrum Phos 30:* Fever accompanied by throbbing head. Take one dose as necessary.

*Gelsemium 30:* Drowsy, aching, chilly, heavy, no thirst. Take one dose as necessary.

*Merc Sol 30:* Sweating, worse at night, offensive smell in room, thirsty. Take one dose of the 30th potency twice a day for three days.

*Pulsatilla 30:* Fevers in children. Child becomes clingy. Changeable moods, thirstless, desires fresh air. Take one dose of the 30th potency twice a day for three days.

AROMATHERAPY

*Roman Chamomile, Lavender:* Add a few drops of one to the bath or sponge the patient down from a bowl of water with two to three drops of the oil added.

*Eucalyptus:* Add a few drops of water and spray around the room to disinfect it.

# FLATULENCE

Gas in the stomach and intestines caused by the intake of air during eating or drinking, or undigested food fermenting; often accompanied by a bloated feeling, abdominal pain, belching and passing gas.

Avoid foods that you know cause this feeling, also don't eat or drink when you are overtired, anxious or angry. Eat slowly, chewing each mouthful well before swallowing.

HERBS

*Aniseed, Caraway, Fennel, Peppermint:* Any of the above may be taken on their own, or combined and made into an infusion using one teaspoon per cup. Leave to stand for ten minutes, strain and drink after meals.

## HOMŒOPATHY

*Carbo Veg or 30:* One dose as required for repeated belching, bloated sensation in abdomen, belching alleviates the discomfort. Useful in elderly people.

*China 6 or 30:* One dose when stomach feels full of gas, distention, passing wind does not ameliorate.

*Lycopodium 6 or 30:* One dose with fullness even after light eating; rumbling and gurgling in abdomen.

*Mag Phos 6:* One dose when required for flatulence with much belching of gas and crampy pains.

## AROMATHERAPY

*Aniseed, Coriander, Fennel, Peppermint:* Any of the above oils will help relieve flatulence. Two to three drops diluted in a light vegetable oil base and lightly massaged over the abdomen.

# FLU
(See: INFLUENZA.)

# FRACTURES

It is often difficult to tell if a bone is broken — an X-ray will be needed, and the bone set rigid in plaster to allow it to heal. The most common sites of fractures are the wrist, ankle and the collar bone. Old people are more prone to fractures if their bones are weakened. The following remedies will promote healing of the bones.

(See also: ACCIDENTS.)

## HERBS

*Alfalfa, Comfrey, Horsetail:* These herbs will help the bones to heal faster by promoting collagen formation. Make an infusion or use the tinctures and take three times daily for up to six weeks.

*Comfrey Oil or Ointment:* This may be applied externally.

HOMŒOPATHY

*Arnica 30 or 200:* One or two doses a day for three to five days for shock with bruising, swelling and tenderness.

*Eupatorium Perf 30:* For aching pain in bones. One dose two times a day for one or two weeks.

*Hypericum 200:* One dose a day for three days for agonizing pain involving nerves.

*Symphytum 6 or 30:* Twice daily promotes healing and union of bones. Take for up to three weeks.

AROMATHERAPY

*Lavender, Rosemary, Thyme:* Combine 1% of each in a bottle of *Comfrey* oil or vegetable base oil and gently massage morning and night to promote healing and help with the aching.


# FUNGAL INFECTION
(See: ATHLETE'S FOOT, THRUSH.)

# G

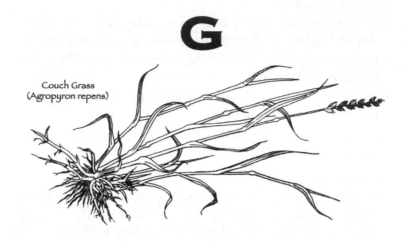

Couch Grass
(Agropyron repens)

## GASTRITIS

An inflammation of the lining of the stomach, often caused by poor diet, irritants like tobacco and alcohol, and hurried meals. A stressful lifestyle could also be a major contributory factor. The symptoms are heartburn, acidic risings and pain in the abdomen. Only easily digested foods should be eaten. It may be useful to visit a naturopath for dietary advice.

Occasional gastric symptoms will be felt by most people sometimes, but if the problem is more persistent or constitutes a marked change from a previously stable pattern, professional advice should be sought, because gastritis can be an early symptom of several different digestive diseases.

(See also: INDIGESTION)

### HERBS

*Marshmallow Leaves, Meadowsweet, Plantain:* Combine in equal parts and make an infusion using one teaspoon of herbs to a cupful of boiling water. Drink three cups a day.

*Slippery Elm:* A light and soothing nutritional food. Stir a teaspoon of the powdered herb into a little warm water to make a paste, top up the cup with warm water, and drink after each meal, or three times a day.

HOMŒOPATHY

*Kali Mur 6X:* Indigestion from fatty or rich food. Nausea. Stomach feels heavy. Ameliorated by a cold drink. One dose every few hours when required.

*Nat Carb 6:* Weak digestion, aggravated by slight errors in the diet. Acidity and belching. Heartburn after fatty food. One dose every few hours as necessary.

*Nat Phos 6X:* Ailments from excess acidity. Sour eructations. One dose every few hours as required.

*Nux Vom 6:* Waterbrash, nausea and sour eructations. Pain in the stomach, back and chest. Aggravated by rich food, stimulants and alcohol. One dose every two to three hours as necessary.

*Pulsatilla 6:* Aggravated by fat and rich food. Nausea and heartburn with a bad taste in the mouth. Thirstlessness. Stomach feels deranged and heavy. One dose every few hours as necessary.

AROMATHERAPY

*Chamomile, Marjoram, Orange:* Choose one of the above oils. Add a few drops to a little vegetable oil and massage over the abdomen, or add two or three drops of one of the oils to a warm bath.

## GASTROENTERITIS

Inflammation of stomach and intestines, which produces symptoms such as abdominal pain, vomiting and diarrhoea. This results from a variety of causes, such as viral, e.g. gastric 'flu, food or metal poisoning and infections. Care must be taken that the person does not become dehydrated and that the normal electrolyte balance of the body is maintained. In a young child failure to hold down clear fluids, drowsiness, disinterest in fluids and decreased passage of urine are all warning signs of the need for urgent professional advice.

Following the first symptoms of gastroenteritis the stomach should be rested for the first eight hours with only sips of water being taken; after the first eight hours, to prevent dehydration, plenty of fluids should be taken, possibly with a pinch of salt and sugar added. After twenty-four hours plain, light food may be introduced. If symptoms are not relieved by the following remedies after twenty-four hours, or before that time in young children, seek immediate medical aid. (See also: DIARRHOEA.)

## HERBS

*Chamomile, Marshmallow Root, Meadowsweet:* Make an infusion using a heaped teaspoon of the combined herbs to a cupful of water and stand for ten minutes. Drink a cupful three times a day to soothe the digestive system.

*Fenugreek:* Add two teaspoons of crushed seeds to a cupful of boiling water and simmer for 15 minutes. Drink three times a day to help eliminate the infection and soothe the digestive system.

*Slippery Elm:* A light and soothing nutritious food. This may be introduced before other more solid food can be tolerated. Stir a teaspoon of the herb into a little warm water to make a paste, top up the cup with warm water, and drink three times a day.

## HOMŒOPATHY

*Ars Alb 30:* Violent vomiting and diarrhoea accompanied with abdominal pains. Chilly, restless, exhausted, fearful and feverish. Burning sensations. Aggravated at night and by eating. One dose three times a day for three days.

*Belladonna 30:* Acute violent throbbing pains in the stomach accompanied with fever. Dosage as for *Ars Alb*

*Bryonia 30:* Nausea with vomiting and abdominal pain. Pain worse when moving and in the morning. Feels irritable. Better when lying on the stomach. Thirsty with dry mouth. Dosage as for *Ars Alb*.

*Colocynth 30:* Severe abdominal pains with vomiting and diarrhoea. Doubles up with the pain and holds the stomach because pressure and warmth bring relief. Feels better after a stool. Dosage as for *Ars Alb*.

*Ipecac 30:* Persistent nausea with vomiting, the nausea continues even after vomiting. Patient has a clean tongue. Vomit and stool contains mucous. Dosage as for *Ars Alb*.

*Mag Phos 30:* Crampy abdominal pains ameliorated by pressure and warmth. Dosage as for *Ars Alb*.

*Nux Vom 30:* Vomiting and retching. Back aches. Chilly, irritable patient. Patient much relieved after vomiting. Dosage as for *Ars Alb*.

*Phosphorus 30:* Burning pain in the stomach with vomiting. Thirst for cold drinks that are vomited soon after swallowing. Better after sleep. Dosage as for *Ars Alb*.

*Podophyllum 30:* Profuse, smelly diarrhoea. Dosage as for *Ars Alb*.

*Pulsatilla 30:* Nausea and diarrhoea. Worse at night, and worse in a warm room. Thirstless, craves open air. Children become clingy and weepy. Dosage as for *Ars Alb*.

*Veratrum Alb 30:* Cramping pains in the abdomen followed by profuse diarrhoea. Patient covered in cold sweat. Craves cold water and refreshing things which aggravate. Dosage as for *Ars Alb*.

AROMATHERAPY

*Cypress, Chamomile:* Add a few drops to a vegetable oil base and lightly massage onto the abdomen.

*Thyme:* This may be sprayed in the room as a disinfectant.


# GINGIVITIS

An infection of the surface tissues of the gums, found in association with certain bacteria, which an increase in oral hygiene will help eliminate. Eating refined foods and sugar are contributary causes. This condition must not be neglected as it can lead to weakening of the gums and eventual loss of teeth.

HERBS

*Echinacea, Myrrh:* Combine and use one teaspoon of each herb; simmer for ten minutes. Strain and allow to cool; use as a mouthwash. The above may be used in tincture form; dilute five drops of each in a glass of warm water and use as a mouthwash.

*Calendula:* A freshly made infusion can be 'swilled and swallowed' or add a couple of drops of tincture to warm water and use as a mouthwash.

AROMATHERAPY

*Lavender, Myrrh:* Add three drops of each to warm boiled water. Use as a mouthwash at least twice a day.

# GOUT

A build-up of uric acid around one or two joints, most commonly the big toe, that become swollen and excruciatingly painful.

Diet will be of great importance in the treatment of gout: avoid rich, fatty foods; stimulants including spices, tobacco and alcohol. This condition does have an hereditary factor.

A qualified practitioner should be consulted, and the following remedies may be used as an adjunct to their treatment, with their approval. As well as the three therapies of herbalism, homœopathy, and aromatherapy, we particularly recommend acupuncture and naturopathy for the treatment of gout.

HERBS

*Celery Seed, Dandelion Leaves, Meadowsweet, Nettle, Sarsaparilla, White Willow:* Combine the herbs in equal parts. Make an infusion using one teaspoon of herbs to a cupful of boiling water, stand for ten minutes, strain. Drink a cupful of infusion, or use the tinctures three times a day for up to six weeks.

*Cabbage Leaf:* A freshly made *Cabbage Leaf* poultice will bring immediate relief.

## HOMŒOPATHY

The following remedies may alleviate an acute attack of gout, to prevent a recurrence constitutional treatment from a qualified practitioner will be required.

*Belladonna 30:* The joint is very red, hot and inflamed. Pulsating or throbbing pain. Take one dose every six hours.

*Colchicum 30:* Joint is excruciatingly tender with shooting and tearing pains. One dose every six hours.

*Nat Phos 6X, Nat Sulph 6X:* These tissue salts will encourage the body to eliminate acid deposits more effectively. Take one of each morning and evening for ten days.

## AROMATHERAPY

*Benzoin, Juniper, Rosemary:* Regular massage with a combination of these oils will help with the pain and encourage elimination of the acid deposits. Add a few drops of each to a light vegetable oil base and gently massage the area surrounding the painful joint. Do not attempt massage during an acute attack but rather use the oils in a compress.

# H

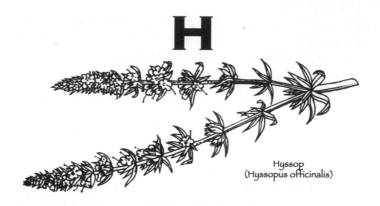

Hyssop
(Hyssopus officinalis)

## HAEMORRHOIDS

Haemorrhoids (or piles) are distended veins in the rectal area, often painless, but they may rupture, bleed, itch or cause pain. Frequent causes are constipation, liver congestion and pregnancy. There is also a hereditary factor. This is a common complaint that can be helped considerably by correct treatment. However, other more serious forms of rectal bleeding may mimic or co-exist with haemorrhoids, consult a physician for a diagnosis.

If constipation is a causative factor, then a naturopath should be consulted for advice on diet. Rutin tablets (a bioflavonoid) may be added to the diet (or eat more buckwheat) as this will strengthen the capillary walls.

(See also: VARICOSE VEINS.)

### HERBS

*Dandelion Root, Horse Chestnut, Stone Root, Yarrow:* Make an infusion using a heaped teaspoon to a cup of boiling water and stand for ten minutes before straining, or use the tinctures. Drink a cupful three times a day.

*Pilewort:* An ointment may be made from this herb to apply externally.

*Witchazel:* Distilled *Witchazel* may be diluted in water and applied externally to soothe inflammation and relieve itching.

HOMŒOPATHY

*Arnica 6 or 30:* Painful haemorrhoids caused by childbirth or over-straining. Bruised sensation. One 30 a day for three days, or one 6 three times a day for five days.

*Calc Fluor 6X:* Tendency to lax fibres, varicose veins and piles. Will tone up the elastic tissues. One dose morning and night for ten days.

*Collinsonia 6 or 30:* Sensation of sharp sticks in the rectum. Painful, bleeding and protruding piles with constipation. One 30 potency a day for three days, or one 6 three times a day for five days.

*Hamamelis 6 or 30:* Piles, bleeding profusely, with soreness and a bruised feeling. Tendency to varicose veins and piles, one 30 potency a day for three days, or one 6 three times a day for five days.

*Nit Ac 6 or 30:* Painful, easily bleeding piles. Prolonged pain after stools. Rectum feels torn. One 30 a day for three days or one 6 potency three times a day for five days.

*Nux Vomica 6 or 30:* Itching piles. Alleviated by cool bathing. Patient is irritable with the pain. One 30 potency a day for three days or one 6 three times a day for five days.

*Sulphur 6 or 30:* Large haemorrhoids that are sore, tender, raw, burn, bleed and smart. One 30 a day for three days or one 6 three times a day for five days.

AROMATHERAPY

*Cypress, Lavender, Myrrh:* Add a few drops of any of the above to a warm bath or apply as a local compress.

# HANGOVERS

An over-indulgence in alcohol puts a great strain on the liver, which attempts to process all the toxins. As so many alcoholic drinks these days are laced with dubious chemicals this will put an added strain on the liver. Obviously people with a weakness in this organ would be well advised to avoid all alcohol.

Symptoms of a hangover include headache, dry mouth, thirst, irritability and nausea. The following remedies will offer relief for an occasional hangover; if these complaints occur regularly then counselling regarding alcoholism tendencies should be considered.

## HERBS

*Balm, Chamomile, Dandelion Leaves, Meadowsweet, Yarrow:* A combination of these herbs will encourage the body to eliminate toxins and be soothing for any headache or nausea. Make an infusion using a heaped teaspoon of the mixed herbs to a cupful of boiling water. Drink a cupful every few hours.

*Milk Thistle:* This is a liver tonic that helps to repair the damage done to the liver by alcohol. Make an infusion or take the tincture three times a day.

## HOMŒOPATHY

*Cocculus 6:* Dizziness and nausea, drowsiness. Especially after excessive drinking of beer. One dose every few hours.

*Nat Phos 6X:* Will relieve symptoms of dehydration. Counteracts acidity (after excessive drinking of wine). One dose every few hours.

*Nat Sulph 6X:* Assists the liver in eliminating toxins. Dull heavy headache. One dose every few hours.

*Nux Vom 30:* Oversensitivity to noise. Irritability, nausea. General effects of over-indulgence of food, alcohol, tobacco or stimulants. One dose every few hours.

## AROMATHERAPY

*Grapefruit, Juniper, Rosemary:* Add one drop of each to a bath oil or shower gel, or add a couple of drops of each to a little vegetable base oil for a massage.

# HAYFEVER

Hayfever is a common complaint, usually a seasonal allergy caused by higher levels of pollen in the air. The usual symptoms which include sneezing, runny or stuffy nose, streaming and itching eyes, are also the symptoms of other allergies like dust, animal fur, etc.

To cure the tendency to hayfever, will require constitutional treatment by an experienced practitioner. The following remedies will help to alleviate discomfort without the unpleasant side effects found with hayfever drug treatment.

(See also: ALLERGIES.)

## HERBS

### INTERNAL

*Elderflower, Eyebright, Hyssop, Nettle:* Combine in equal quantities and make an infusion using one teaspoon per cupful of boiling water, or use the tinctures. Take three times per day.

### EXTERNAL

*Eyebright:* Make an infusion as above, but cool, and then use to bathe the eyes regularly. Or add one to two drops of tincture to a little cooled, boiled water and bathe the eyes.

## HOMŒOPATHY

*Allium Cepa, Euphrasia, Sabadilla 6 or 30:* A combination remedy that may be taken three times a day when hayfever symptoms are present.

*Mixed Pollens 30:* Take twice a week during the hayfever season.

## AROMATHERAPY

*Cypress, Eucalyptus, Juniper:* Put two drops of each in a bowl of hot water and use as a steam inhalation.

## HEADACHES

Nearly everyone has a headache at one time or another as there are so many causes. They may be a sign that one is over-stressed, or they may result from toxins, e.g. tobacco, alcohol, etc., or they may be associated with a cold, fever, PMT, or caused by structural conditions such as a neck injury or bad posture. Obviously, if headaches are very severe or persist, or result from an injury, medical advice must be sought immediately, because there are other more serious causes of headaches.

Alexander Technique will be useful if bad posture is a causative factor; acupuncture, homœopathy and other therapies will help as constitutional treatment for recurrent headaches. For the occasional headache with an obvious, non-serious cause, the following remedies will be helpful,

(See also: HANGOVERS, MIGRAINE, SUNSTROKE.)

HERBS

*Balm, Meadowsweet, Peppermint, Rosemary, Vervain:*
  Combine, make an infusion using a heaped teaspoon to a cupful of boiling water, and drink a cup every few hours. Also consider the following herbs by looking them up in a herbal repertory: *Chamomile, Lavender, Lime Flowers, Skullcap, White Willow, Wood Betony.*

HOMŒOPATHY

*Aconite 30:* Sudden violent headache, worse in the evening. Comes on after taking a cold or a fright.

*Arnica 30:* Brought on by a fall or injury. Bruised feeling in head.

*Belladonna 30:* Throbbing pain. Head feels hot. Dilated pupils.

*Bryonia 30:* Bursting, heavy, crushing, splitting headache. Worse for any movement, better lying still.

*Calc Phos, Kali Phos, Mag Phos 6X:* Headaches from stress, strain and overworking. One dose every two hours.

*Gelsemium 6 or 30:* Begins at the back of the neck. Heavy, dull headache. Associated with fluey symptoms or apprehension.

*Iris 30:* Aches begin with blurring of vision. Sick headaches. Shooting pain in temples. Tired headache after mental work.

*Kali Bich 30:* Preceded by visual disturbances. Aching in the sinuses. Pain as of a solid block in the forehead. Catarrhal headaches.

*Nux Vomica 30:* Irritable headache brought on by over-indulgence in coffee, alcohol, etc., or by over-studying. Overall sick feeling.

*Pulsatilla 30:* Headache with nausea and gastric or menstrual disturbances. Better by walking in open air. Miserable and weepy.

AROMATHERAPY

*Bergamot, Chamomile, Eucalyptus, Peppermint, Rosemary:* Choose from the above, dilute in vegetable oil and massage into the feet to draw the tension away from the head. Alternatively, add a few drops to a warm bath

*Lavender:* Massage one drop into each temple.


# HIGH BLOOD PRESSURE (HYPERTENSION)

There are many factors involved in this common problem, and prevention is much better than cure. A holistic practitioner should be consulted to look into the main contributing aspects in each case. Ongoing supervision is crucial: once recognised, regular checks over an indefinite period should be arranged with a physician. Many people need to continue lifelong with treatment in order to prevent stroke, kidney disease or heart failure.

A diet rich in animal fats, salt and simple sugars should be avoided, as should smoking and alcohol consumption. A high-stress lifestyle is also a predisposing factor. Sometimes the problem is hereditary.

## HERBS

If taking hypertension drugs, a qualified herbalist must be consulted before trying herbal treatment.

*Lime Flowers, Motherwort, Yarrow:* This mixture may be helpful for mild cases. Combine the herbs and make an infusion using one heaped teaspoon of herbs to a cupful of boiling water and stand for ten minutes before straining. Drink a cupful twice daily for up to six weeks.

*Hawthorn:* Improves the circulation and strengthens the heart. Take an infusion or tincture three times a day. This may need to be taken for two to three months for noticeable benefit to be experienced.

## HOMŒOPATHY

Constitutional treatment is advised.

## AROMATHERAPY

Most benefit will be received from regular massage by an experienced aromatherapist.

*Clary Sage, Lavender, Melissa, Ylang Ylang:* Regular massage or baths containing a few drops of one of these oils may be tried.

## BACH FLOWER REMEDIES

We suggest that you look into the use of Bach flower remedies to help with the stress-induced factor of this problem.

# HYPERACTIVITY

Hyperactivity is a syndrome marked by sleeplessness, restlessness and aggressive behaviour. It is not easy to diagnose because the problem varies a lot in degrees, but it does seem to be an increasing problem, particularly in children. Recent research suggests that allergies, food additives, vaccinations and pollution are primary factors to consider; however emotional upset due to family dynamics may also be very significant.

Constitutional treatment by a holistic practitioner is strongly recommended.

## AROMATHERAPY

*Lavender, Mandarin, Rose:* These oils have all been used successfully to calm hyperactivity, and are safe to use with children. Choose one or two and dilute to use as a massage oil or in the bath. They may also be used in a diffuser to create a calming atmosphere.

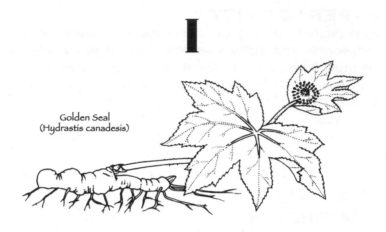

Golden Seal
(Hydrastis canadesis)

## IMPETIGO

A highly contagious infection often contracted from animals; appearing as sores, most commonly on the hands or face, and may include other symptoms such as loss of appetite, nausea, headache and swelling. Scrupulous hygiene is essential to avoid infection and infecting others.

### HERBS

EXTERNAL

*Echinacea, Golden Seal (half), Marigold, Myrrh:* Combine and make a decoction or use the diluted tinctures and bathe regularly.

INTERNAL

*Blue Flag Root, Echinacea, Figwort, Yellow Dock:* Use equal parts, make a decoction or use tinctures and drink three times daily.

### HOMŒOPATHY

*Ant. Crude 6:* Oozing eruptions with thick yellow crusts. Worse on face; individual sores joining together. Looks worse after bathing. Three doses a day for ten days.

*Ars Alb 6:* Sores bleed, with burning pains and rawness,

better from warmth. Exudes a thin watery fluid. Three doses a day for ten days.

*Graphites 6:* Scabby oozing eruptions with sticky discharge. Three doses a day for ten days.

*Merc Sol 6:* Deep open sores with yellowish crusts exuding offensive smelling pus. Three doses a day for ten days.

*Rhus Tox 6:* Extremely itchy and burning sores, blister-like eruptions. Three doses a day for ten days.

AROMATHERAPY

*Myrrh, Tea Tree:* Add three drops of each to an eggcupful of warm water. Apply using cotton wool twice a day.

# INCONTINENCE

This is most common in the elderly, and the chronically sick. If there is no organic problem involved other than loss of control in the sphincter muscle of the bladder, or nervous debility, the following suggestions may be helpful. (See also: BEDWETTING.)

HERBS

*Agrimony, Bayberry, Horsetail:* Make an infusion of two parts *Horsetail* to one part *Agrimony* and *Bayberry* and drink a cupful two or three times daily as a tonic for the urinary system.

HOMŒOPATHY

*Causticum 30:* Bedwetting during first sleep at night. Stress incontinence. Paralysis and weakness of bladder. No sensation in urethra when passing urine. Two doses eight hours apart. May be repeated after six weeks.

*Equisetum 6:* Habitual bedwetting with fullness and distension in bladder. Dribbling urine in the elderly. One dose morning and night for ten days.

*Sepia 30:* Loss of tone of pelvic area and sphincter muscles. Stress incontinence after labour. Two doses eight hours apart. May be repeated after six weeks.

## INDIGESTION

The digestive system may be upset by the intake of rich food, or by the person eating when feeling stressful or tense, or due to fast or irregular eating. The symptoms include heartburn, nausea, flatulence and general discomfort in the stomach region. Occasional dyspeptic symptoms will be felt by most people sometimes, but if the problem is more persistent or constitutes a marked change from a previously stable pattern, professional advice should be sought, because indigestion can be an early symptom of several different digestive diseases. (See also: GASTRITIS.)

HERBS

*Aniseed, Cardamon, Fennel:* A few of any of these seeds chewed after a meal will help with indigestion.

*Balm, Peppermint, Vervain:* A tea made from any of these will be soothing for the digestive system. Drink after a meal.

*Meadowsweet:* Combine this with any of the teas mentioned above if symptoms of acidity are also present.

HOMŒOPATHY

*Ars Alb 6 or 30:* Irritable stomach. Burning in stomach area. Great thirst for hot drinks. Anxious, restless patient. One every few hours.

*Carbo Veg 6 or 30:* Distension and heaviness. Sour, disordered stomach. Flatulence, belching, heartburn and waterbrash. All food turns to wind. Particularly useful in elderly patients. Two or three doses four hours apart.

*Kali Mur 6X:* Heavy feeling. Coated, white tongue. Indigestion after rich, fatty food. One dose every few hours.

*Nat Phos 6X:* Sour risings, heartburn. Liverish symptoms. Acidity. One dose every few hours.

*Nux Vom 6 or 30:* Heartburn, belching. Weight and pain in stomach. Brought on by over-indulgence of food and drink. Irritable. One dose every few hours as necessary.

*Pulsatilla 6 or 30:* From eating fatty food. Nausea. Feeling of distension. Unpleasant taste in the mouth. Better in fresh air. Thirstless. One dose every few hours.

AROMATHERAPY

*Cardamon, Fennel, Peppermint:* Add a few drops of the above to a vegetable based oil and massage into the stomach area.


## INFLUENZA

Influenza commonly called 'flu' is an acute infection of the respiratory tract similar to colds, but more severe, and accompanied by symptoms like fever, aches and coughs. Different strains will produce different symptoms, e.g., sore throat, nausea, and these should be treated specifically. Flu normally lasts between two and five days, but more serious complications may develop, particularly in the elderly. Persons not responding to treatment should be referred to a practitioner.

It seems that an increasing trend with 'flu' is to leave the person debilitated and depressed.

(See also: COLDS, CONVALESCENCE.)

HERBS

*Elderberry:* An herb with effective anti-viral properties to promote recovery. Also suitable for children. Add 1ml of tincture to hot water or to the infusion below and take three times a day.

*Elderflower, Peppermint, Yarrow:* A general mixture for feverish flu symptoms. Combine, infuse, or use the tinctures and take several times a day. The following herbs may also be added to this mixture.

*Echinacea:* If symptoms linger.

*Pleurisy Root:* If a cough is present.

*Red Sage:* If accompanied by a sore throat.

*Vervain:* If accompanied by depression.

HOMŒOPATHY

*Aconite 30:* Sudden onset with fever. Dry, painful cough. Restlessness and anxiety; symptoms develop after exposure to cold winds. Two doses a day on first day or two of symptoms.

*Ars Alb30:* Shivering, restlessness, anxiety; loss of appetite; desires hot drinks; worse from cold drinks. Burning sensations; worse after midnight. Feels very chilly. Take three doses a day.

*Bryonia 30:* Worse with movement; desire to be alone; irritable; dry and thirsty, painful cough, throat and chest. Take three doses a day.

*Eupatorium Perf 30:* Intense aching; bursting headache; soreness of eyeballs. Hacking cough and hoarseness; nausea; marked thirst. Take three doses a day.

*Gelsemium 30:* Heaviness, and drowsy patient; chills up and down the spine. Aching in limbs and head. Little thirst. General flu symptoms. Take three doses a day.

*Rhus Tox 30:* Extremely restlessness, muscles stiff and aching. Chill; worse after getting cold or wet. Thirsty, hoarseness. Take three doses a day.

AROMATHERAPY

*Lavender, Ravensara, Rosemary:* Dilute in suitable vegetable oil base and massage into chest and aching limbs.

*Eucalyptus, Tea Tree:* Add a few drops to hot water. Use as a steam inhalation for congestion, or add to a burner.

# INSOMNIA

Sleeplessness may be a short-term or long-term problem. The amount of sleep needed will vary from person to person, and for the same person at different stages of their life. Short-term sleeplessness may be brought about by anxiety, fear, stress or excitement. Most people will suffer the odd sleepless night at some time; the problem is that sleeplessness can become rather a habit, and anxiety will develop around not being able to sleep which may become self-perpetuating. Sleep disorders such as early morning waking, if accompanied by dark moods, can indicate an underlying depression which may need professional help. The following remedies will be useful to break the habit, but for chronic insomniacs constitutional treatment by a qualified practitioner will be necessary.

A useful exercise if the mind is full of thoughts and unresolved problems is to mentally work backwards through the day going over everything you have done without becoming attached to any one issue. Stimulating foods and drinks, and eating late at night can all be aggravating factors, and should be avoided.

## HERBS

*Balm, Chamomile, Lime Flowers, Orange Blossom, Passiflora:* A pleasant tasting relaxing bedtime drink.

*SKullcap, Vervain:* Add these to the above mixture if nervous tension is present.

*Vulerian:* Add if the mixture needs to be stronger, e.g. if pain is present. This particular herb does not suit everybody, and may become habit-forming, so do not use too frequently.

## HOMŒOPATHY

*Aconite 30:* Anxiety with restlessness and fear. Anxious dreams. Try one dose and only repeat if necessary.

*Arnica 30:* Sleeplessness due to being overtired, after overworking, or due to shock. Body aches and the bed feels too hard. One dose as required.

*Coffea 6 or 30:* Thoughts racing around the mind. Sleeplessness due to anxiety and agitation. One dose as required.

*Kali Phos 6X:* Nervous tension, habitual sleeplessness. Take one a night for ten nights; this remedy should begin to work after the second or third night.

*Kali Phos, Mag Phos, Nat Phos 6X:* Aids sleep after stress. Insomnia from being under strain and overwrought. Two or three doses at 30 minute intervals.

*Nux Vomica 30:* Person falls asleep in the evening, but wakes too early and still feels tired when it is time to get up. Irritability. Indigestion. Try one dose and do not repeat for several weeks.

## AROMATHERAPY

*Chamomile, Lavender, Neroli:* Add a few drops of the above mixture to a warm bath.

*Lavender:* Put a couple of drops on a piece of cotton wool and place on the pillow.

## BACH FLOWER REMEDIES

The following may be useful when dealing with the emotional contributory factors.

*Olive:* Exhaustion, tired but sleepless. Needing sleep.

*Vervain:* Over-straining, over-enthusiasm.

*White Chestnut:* Persistent and racing worries and troubles.

# J

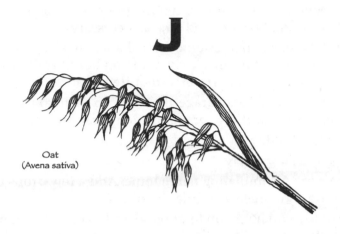

Oat
(Avena sativa)

## JET LAG

There are a few remedies which may ease the discomfort often felt during or after travelling by air. Symptoms are due to a combination of sitting or sleeping for long periods of time where the circulation is impeded, the body struggling to become accustomed to the time changes and change of sleep patterns and, thirdly, to the changing pressure in the aircraft. Avoid alcohol as this will add to the dehydration resulting from the pressure changes; drink plenty of spring water.

### HERBS

*Oat Tincture:* A mildly diuretic nervine tincture to be taken during the flight to ease swelling in the feet and aid relaxation. Ten drops in water every six hours.

*Kola, Oat, Rosemary Tinctures:* This mixture will stimulate and tonify the nervous system and help you to adjust on arrival. Buy as a mixture and take ten drops in water every four to six hours during the flight.

### HOMŒOPATHY

*Arnica 30:* One dose for every four hours of flight time, plus one dose on arrival. Helps with exhaustion and trauma of jet lag and long flights.

*Kali Mur 6 or 30:* Earache due to pressure changes. One dose before take-off, and take as necessary.

*Kali Phos 6X:* A nerve tonic for exhaustion, sleeplessness and tension. Take every six hours on board and for two to three days after arrival as required.

*Nat Mur 6X:* To encourage the body to maintain correct water distribution, prevents dehydration. One dose every four hours.

AROMATHERAPY

*Rosemary:* A stimulating nerve tonic. Add a few drops to a tissue and inhale at regular intervals.

*Lavender:* Will help you to unwind and sleep at the appropriate time. Add to the bath the evening of arrival, or add a few drops to a tissue and place on the pillow at bedtime.

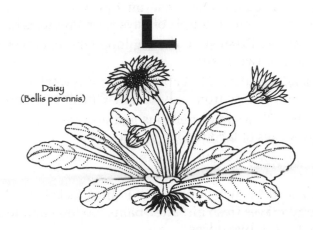

L

Daisy
(Bellis perennis)

## LABOUR

The progress of the birth of a child, of which there are three stages: (1) dilatation of the cervix; (2) the passage of the foetus through the canal, and the birth; and (3) from the birth of the child to the expulsion of the placenta.

Childbirth is a natural process; there are many books available to help prepare yourself and your environment. The following remedies may complement the aid and advice of a competent midwife and/or doctor. It is advisable to be under the guidance of a qualified practitioner during pregnancy, and they should be able to advise you on your labour.

(See also: PREGNANCY.)

### HERBS

*Raspberry Leaf, Squaw Vine:* Can be drunk during the last three months of pregnancy to help facilitate an easier labour. Combine and make an infusion or take the tinctures.

### HOMŒOPATHY

*Aconite 30 or 200:* Fear, shock, after pains with fear and restlessness. One or two doses.

*Arnica 30 or 200:* Bruising and symptoms of over-exhaustion after labour. One dose on first going into labour, and one a day for a couple of days after. Promotes healing.

*Carbo Veg 30:* Exhaustion during long labour, craves fresh air. One or two doses.

*Caulophyllum 30 or 200:* Labour pains are weak or irregular, or may cease from exhaustion. One or two doses.

*Gelsemium 30:* Rigid or nervous fear and trembling during early stages of labour. One or two doses.

*Mag Phos 30:* Shooting, stabbing after-pains. One or two doses.

*Pulsatilla 30:* Weak labour pains. Patient feels irritable and weepy, craves fresh air; after-pains too long and too violent. One or two doses.

AROMATHERAPY

*Clary Sage:* Can be burned or sprayed in the room to freshen it.

*Jasmine:* To help with the pain of childbirth; massaged on the lower back in a base of vegetable oil.

*Rose:* Is cooling and soothing. Can be used diluted in a vegetable base oil for massage.

BACH FLOWER REMEDIES

*Five Flower Remedy:* If the labour is long and exhausting, and if there is fear or panic involved. Take as necessary.


# LABOUR (POST)

The following remedies may be helpful to use after labour as indicated.

HERBS

EXTERNAL

*Comfrey, Horsetail, Marigold, St John's Wort:* Add one heaped tablespoonful to a pint of water. Leave to infuse and pour into a warm bath for a soothing and healing effect to the perineum.

INTERNAL

*Raspberry Leaf, Squaw Vine:* Encourages the uterus to return back to normal. Make an infusion using a heaped teaspoon to a cup of boiling water. Drink two times daily for two or three weeks.

*Blue Cohosh:* If after-pains are present. Make a docoction or use the tincture and drink three times a day.

*Alfalfa, Nettle:* If exhaustion is present. Make an infusion and drink a cupful twice daily.

HOMŒOPATHY

*Bellis Perennis 30:* Painful, sensitive feeling in genital organs after forceps delivery, or pain in abdomen after Caesarian birth. Two doses a day for three days.

*Hypericum 30:* To heal episiotomy or lacerations during forceps delivery. Two doses a day for four days.

*Chamomilla 30:* Severe after-pains, patient is acutely sensitive to pain, feels irritable. Two or three doses over two days.

*Mag Phos 30:* Spasmodic shooting after-pains. Two or three doses over two days.

AROMATHERAPY

*Lavender:* For soothing baths after childbirth, add four drops to a warm bath.


# LICE

The parasite concerned in head lice (also known as pediculosis) is Pediculus humanus capitis. The first sign is often itching, the severity of which depends on the immune response to the salivary antigens of the louse. The affected hairs become lustreless and dry, but the diagnosis is made by finding the lice, or more often oval-lidded white capsules (egg cases), known as 'nits', firmly attached to the hair shaft.

Head lice have always been a major problem in schools, and other places where people congregate together.

Anyone can get head lice and getting them bears no relation to how frequently you wash your hair. Fortunately, a number of essential oils are effective in removing head lice. It is advisable to treat the whole family as lice are very easily passed on. To prevent re-infestation any lice and eggs must be removed from collars, hats, scarves and bedding. Wash everything that can be washed in soap powder. A strong decoction of *Quassia* chips (see below) may be used to sponge down pillows, mattresses, coat collars and hoods etc.

## HERBS
*Quassia:* A decoction of this insect-repelling herb may be used as the final rinse when washing the hair to help prevent re-infestation. This may be used in conjunction with the aromatherapy suggestions.

## AROMATHERAPY
*Cedarwood, Lavender, Rosemary, Tea Tree:* Add twenty drops of each essential oil to 100ml of a vegetable base oil, such as almond or sunflower oil. Massage 10-15ml (depending on the length of the hair) very thoroughly into the hair and scalp and comb through the hair. Cover the head and leave on for at least four hours, before washing out with shampoo. Comb through the hair with a fine-toothed comb to remove lice and eggs. Repeat the process after forty-eight hours and once more after eight days to prevent reinfestation.

# LIVER PROBLEMS
The liver is the largest organ of the body, and is involved either directly or indirectly in all physiological processes. One of its important functions is in the eliminating process of toxins, and thus a diet including chemicals, additives, alcohol or drugs will place strain on the liver. It is often helpful to aid the liver with a cleansing diet and purifying herbs, even if no symptoms of liver disease are present; and most spring cleansing remedies and diets

contain liver detoxifiers. There are many symptoms of liver disease; including constipation, nausea, sluggishness, irritability, poor skin, pain in the liver region and dull headaches. If you suspect there is any actual disease of the liver, consult a qualified practitioner. Avoid fatty, rich foods, alcohol and coffee. The following remedies will be cleansing and tonifying.

HERBS

*Burdock, Dandelion:* A traditional cleansing tonic for the liver. Combine equal quantities and make an infusion using one teaspoon per cup. Drink three cups per day.

*Milk Thistle:* Protects and helps to repair damage to the liver. Take the infusion or tincture three times a day for up to six weeks.

HOMŒOPATHY

*Nat Phos 6X:* Liverishness, acidity, poor digestion, sour risings. Twice a day for ten days.

*Nat Sulph 6X:* Heaviness, sluggishness, bilious vomiting. Twice a day for ten days.

AROMATHERAPY

*Grapefruit, Juniper, Rosemary:* These oils will help detoxify the liver. Use in a massage base oil or add to a warm bath.

## LARYNGITIS
(See: SORE THROATS.)

# M

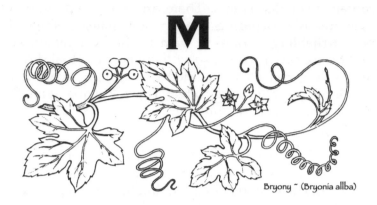

Bryony ~ (Bryonia allba)

## MASTITIS

Inflammation of the breasts. This may be due to infection (most common when breastfeeding), growths, or part of a premenstrual picture, and thus may be either acute or of a chronic nature. If symptoms are persistent, a qualified practitioner must be seen for a diagnosis and treatment. For pre-menstrual mastitis, try *Evening Primrose Oil* capsules, two a day for ten days before each period. It is advisable for all women to perform monthly self-examination so that any deviation from the norm can be noted and checked out by a competent practitioner.

There is some evidence that caffeine may aggravate the tendency to cystic growth formation in the breasts, and thus tea and coffee should be avoided. The following remedies may be tried for acute mastitis. If symptoms persist consult medical advice. If you are breastfeeding and develop mastitis with a fever urgent medical advice should be sought.

(See also: BREASTFEEDING.)

HERBS

EXTERNAL

*Cabbage:* Crush a cabbage leaf with a rolling pin and place over the inflamed breast. Hold in place with your bra.

*Comfrey, Marshmallow, Slippery Elm:* These herbs can be used to make a soothing poultice for acute mastitis.

INTERNAL

*Chamomile, Echinacea, Marigold, Red Clover:* Combine, make an infusion or use the tinctures and take three times a day for acute inflammation.

HOMŒOPATHY

*Belladonna 30:* Pain, throbbing and redness in breast. Streaks radiate from the nipple. Breast feels heavy and hard. One dose every few hours until pain diminishes.

*Bryonia 30:* Breast hot, painful and hard. Cannot bear touch or movement. Better for hard pressure or keeping still. Undue engorgement of breasts. One dose every few hours until improvement occurs.

*Phytolacca 30:* Heavy, stony hard, swollen or tender breasts, pain during breastfeeding or worse before menses. Nipples cracked and sensitive. One dose every few hours until improvement occurs.

AROMATHERAPY

*Chamomile, Geranium, Rose:* Dilute a few drops of each in water. Apply as a soothing and cooling compress.

*Lavender:* This oil diluted in the bath will be soothing. Essential oils are too strong for a baby, so if breastfeeding the breasts must be washed free from the oil before the baby feeds again.

## MEASLES

An infectious disease that prior to immunization was common in children; the incubation period is ten to twelve days. Early symptoms are those of a cold, sore throat, inflamed eyes, cough, rise in temperature, and possibly you may be able to see 'Koplik's spots' (small, white spots on the inside of the cheeks).

The rash appears on about the fourth day on the neck and behind the ears, gradually extending to the rest of the body and extremities. Recovery usually occurs by about the seventh or ninth day. The most infectious period is before the rash appears.

The disease is not usually dangerous, but occasionally complications can develop, usually due to a high fever with dehydration, or breathing difficulties due to chest infection. Very rarely, a more serious complication involving inflammation of the brain tissues — encephalitis — may occur: any unusual drowsiness or irritability should be assessed by a medical practitioner. The eyes may also become sore and inflamed, and the rash may cause distress from itching. If any symptoms are very marked or persistent, seek immediate professional advice. Antibiotics do not have any effect on the virus, so they should not be prescribed unless complications set in.

We do not recommend immunisation against measles because the long-term effects of this are not fully known, and we believe, as with all childhood illnesses, measles provides the opportunity for the child to strengthen his/her vitality and throw off inherited miasmatic tendencies.

General home care should involve bed rest in a darkened room, and during the fever sponging down with tepid water.

## HERBS

### INTERNAL

*Catnip, Chamomile, Echinacea, Elderflowers, Yarrow:* Make an infusion of a combination of these herbs using one teaspoon of herbs to a cupful of boiling water, or use the tinctures. Take three times a day.

### EXTERNAL

*Eyebright:* Make an infusion and when cool, strain and bathe the eyes with the solution to soothe them. Or use one drop of tincture to a little cooled, boiled water.

*Chamomile, Marigold, Marshmallow:* Combine the herbs and make an infusion using one tablespoon of herbs to a pint of boiling water. When cool, strain and use the solution to sponge down the body to cool down fever-ishness and soothe irritation or itching.

## HOMŒOPATHY

*Aconite 30:* For initial stages. Restless, fearful child, high temperature, eyes ache with light. Eyes and nose streaming, hard croupy cough. Give every few hours until improvement occurs.

*Belladonna 30 or 200:* Restless, flushed, high temperature and delirium, sore throat, disturbed by noise, light and movement. One or two doses.

*Bryonia 30:* Use if the rash is slow to appear; accompanied by painful, dry cough; thirsty; irritable; worse from movement. Two or three doses a day.

*Euphrasia 30:* Marked eye symptoms and nasal discharge. Eyes watery, sore and inflamed. Acrid tears, harsh cough, throbbing headache. Two or three doses over two days.

*Kali Bich 30:* Laryngitis with hoarse, brassy cough, cough predominates, earache and nausea, eyes water and eyelids stick together. Two or three doses over two to three days.

*Morbillinum 30:* For cases not responding to treatment, this is the measles nosode. One dose only.

*Pulsatilla 30:* Catarrhal symptoms; profuse lachrymation; cough dry at night, looser in daytime; dry mouth, but seldom thirsty. Two or three doses over two to three days.

## AROMATHERAPY

*Chamomile, Eucalyptus, Lavender:* Dilute a few drops in water and use to sponge down the body.

# MENOPAUSE

A time of transition when the ovaries stop releasing an ovum every month, and the woman is no longer fertile. Menstruation stops because there is no stimulus from the ovaries.

The age of the menopause varies although it is generally

from the middle or later forties. The onset can be gradual with the periods coming less frequently, or it may occur quite suddenly.

Reactions to the menopause seem to depend on the general state of health and on the ability to cope with transition. In physical terms the accompanying changes are due to a readjustment of pituitary and ovarian hormones. The most commonly experienced problematic symptoms are hot flushes, palpitations, nervous irritability, depression and general debility. Many of the symptoms blamed on the menopause are not due to it; and there is a real danger of neglecting other disorders that could and should be treated. Any post menopausal vaginal bleeding should be assessed by a medical practitioner.

This is a time when constitutional treatment, e.g. by an acupuncturist, herbalist or homœopath, and emotional support e.g. from support groups, can make a tremendous difference to making the transition a positive time of change.

Any persistent discomfort, particularly heavy menstrual bleeding for more than two or three periods, and any inter-menstrual bleeding, should be referred to a qualified practitioner. Hormonal replacement will delay the symptoms rather than encourage the body to adjust as well as having the risk of side-effects.

## HERBS

*Agnus Castus, Black Cohosh, Chinese Angelica, Schizandra, St John's Wort:* A useful mixture to help the body make its hormonal adjustments and tonify the reproductive system. Make a decoction or use the tinctures and drink twice a day for six weeks.

*Sage:* This herb is effective at reducing hot flushes. Make an infusion and drink three times daily, or take the tincture. *Sage* may be added to the above mixture.

*Skullcap, Vervain:* Add these herbs if nervousness or depression is marked.

## HOMŒOPATHY
Constitutional treatment by a qualified homœopath can be of great benefit to help with the physical and mental symptoms associated with the menopause.

## AROMATHERAPY
A course of treatment by an experienced aromatherapist who can select oils for your specific needs, will be of most benefit.

*Geranium, Rose:* These oils will help to balance hormones and tone the reproductive system. Apply in a bath or as a massage on a regular basis.

*Cypress:* To relieve hot flushes. Use daily as a massage oil, or dilute in a bath oil base and add to the bath.

## BACH FLOWER REMEDIES
Look through the list in the Appendix to find the remedies needed for your particular symptoms. We especially suggest:

*Impatiens:* Nervous irritability and impatience.

*Olive:* For weakness, weariness and tiredness.

*Walnut:* To help with times of transition and change.


# MENSTRUAL PROBLEMS
Pain, frequency and duration of menses will vary from woman to woman, and for the same woman at different stages of her life, and to a great extent will reflect her general state of health.

Problems may arise due to hormonal, psychological, mechanical damage, cysts, fibroids, tumours, circulatory or nutritional factors. In any case it is important to assess which factors are most significant. Any problem which becomes severely uncomfortable or is persistent should be referred to a qualified practitioner. This is particularly true if inter-menstrual bleeding occurs, or there are any signs of infection, e.g. pain, unpleasant discharge or increased temperature.

The most common menstrual ailment we are asked to treat is painful periods. Pain at the start of a period is vaguely ascribed to reduction of blood-flow by spasm of the uterus, and pain that comes on later to congestion. We suggest that the following remedies may be helpful in treating painful periods, and as tonics for the reproductive system. Periods which cease or become markedly irregular or heavy require constitutional treatment, because this is a longer-term situation that is not really within the scope of self-diagnosis and treatment. (See also: MENOPAUSE, PRE-MENSTRUAL TENSION.)

## HERBS

*Agnus Castus, Chinese Angelica, Motherwort:* Herbs to tonify the reproductive system and balance the hormones. Combine and make an infusion or use the tinctures and drink three times a day for six weeks.

*Chamomile, Cramp Bark, Raspberry Leaves, Valerian, Vervain:* For period pains. Combine tinctures or herbs and drink three times a day when required.

*Lady's Mantle:* Add this herb if bleeding is heavy.

## HOMŒOPATHY

*Aconite 30:* Menses suppressed due to fright, shock or after exposure to cold. One dose at bedtime, and one the following morning.

*Apis 30:* Burning, stinging pains during or before menses. Scanty discharge of blood. Patient is hot and thirstless. One dose every few hours as required.

*Belladonna 30:* Menses early and profuse. Violent bearing down and throbbing pains. Throbbing headache. One dose every few hours as necessary.

*Bryonia 30:* Menses early and profuse. Cutting pains in uterus and breasts. Splitting headache. Everything is worse for motion and better keeping still and applying pressure. One dose every few hours as required.

*Mag Phos 6X or 30:* Cramping, shooting and spasmodic pains. Pains are better for warmth and rubbing. Dissolve one dose under the tongue as required.

## AROMATHERAPY
*Chamomile, Clary Sage, Cypress, Marjoram, Rose:* Choose two or three oils from the above and add a few drops of each to a vegetable oil base and massage into the abdomen to soothe pain. Or add two or three drops of one of the above for a soothing warm bath.

# MIGRAINE
Migraine is distinguished from a headache by its intensity; it is often accompanied by nausea and vision disorders and usually affects one side of the head. The pain is produced by spasm of blood vessels in the brain. The length of the attack varies from a couple of hours to several days. Effective treatment must be constitutional as the causes are so varied. Contributory factors include stress, tension, hormonal cycles in women, congestive disorders, allergic reactions, and a hereditary pre-disposition.

We feel that individuals can go a long way in helping themselves treat this ailment by ascertaining the more profound psychological and physiological reasons why they are the victims, and then as far as possible reducing the factors that stimulate them.

If the migraine attacks are mild or infrequent, here are some remedies to try.

## HERBS
*Balm, Chamomile, Feverfew, Meadowsweet, Rosemary, Wood Betony:* Combine the above herbs, make an infusion and drink up to three cups a day.

*Agnus Castus:* Add this herb if the migraines are usually worse before or during menstruation.

*Scullcap, Valerian:* Add these herbs if nervous tension is present.

## HOMŒOPATHY
*Belladonna 30:* Intense and violent throbbing pains. Sensitive to noise or movement. Pain begins suddenly,

focused on forehead. Headache relieved by sitting down. Two or three doses.

*Bryonia 30:* Worse from movement, relieved by pressure. Heavy, crushing pain may be accompanied by nausea and vomiting. Patient thirsty and irritable.

*Gelsemium 30:* Headaches begin at the back of the head. Pain extends like a band around the head. Dull, heavy headaches, patient feels confused. Better after urination. Two or three doses.

*Iris 30:* Aches begin with blurring of vision. Sick headaches. Shooting pain in temples. Tired headache after mental work.

*Nux Vomica 30:* Headache brought on by overeating or use of stimulants; accompanied by overall sick feeling. Worse for cold air or wind. Worse in morning. Patient very irritable. Two or three doses.

*Pulsatilla 30:* Associated with digestive upsets, menstrual periods or emotional upsets. Pain in forehead accompanied by throbbing. Better from open air. Nausea. Patient feels weepy. Two or three doses.

## AROMATHERAPY

*Coriander, Lavender, Marjoram, Melissa, Peppermint:* Choose one or two of the above. Dilute a few drops in almond oil and massage into the feet to draw tension away from the head or add to the bath.

# MISCARRIAGE

The first symptom of a miscarriage (spontaneous abortion), is bleeding, sometimes accompanied with pain. It is thought that many miscarriages occur as the body's natural way of rejecting an unhealthy foetus. Thus, no form of treatment should be taken to prevent a miscarriage at all costs. However, miscarriage can also be threatened in case of weakness, stress or trauma in the pregnant woman and then the appropriate remedies may be taken to avoid an unnecessary miscarriage.

Plenty of rest is necessary in all cases of threatened miscarriage. Having excluded other causes of bleeding (e.g. ectopic pregnancy), care should be supervised by a competent medical practitioner who should be kept informed of any changes in the patient's condition.

The emotional trauma experienced after a miscarriage can be considerable, and in this case the support of an experienced and caring practitioner would be a helpful adjunct to that of friends and family.

If there is a history of miscarriages, constitutional treatment will be necessary from the outset of pregnancy, or before. Here we can only offer remedies that may help in conjunction with treatment from a qualified holistic practitioner. (See also: PREGNANCY.)

HERBS

For herbs that must be avoided during pregnancy, see PREGNANCY.

*Cramp Bark, Squaw Vine:* A useful uterine tonic to take if a miscarriage is threatening. Combine the herbs, make a decoction by simmering a teaspoon of herbs in a mugful of water for ten minutes, and drink a cupful three times a day. Alternatively combine the tinctures, and take three times a day.

*Skullcap:* If there is considerable stress involved this herb can be added.

HOMŒOPATHY

*Aconite 30 or 200:* Miscarriage threatens suddenly, usually following a fright, shock or trauma. Marked fearfulness and anxiety. One or two doses.

*Arnica 30 or 200:* Miscarriage threatens after an accident or trauma. Haemorrhage following a blow or accident. Haemorrhage after intercourse. One or two doses.

*Chamomilla 30 or 200:* Threatening miscarriage with distressing, contractive pains. Loss of dark blood with the occasional gush of bright red blood. Symptoms may come on after anger. One or two doses.

*Pulsatilla 30 or 200:* Changeable symptoms. Patient is weepy and in need of support. Malposition of foetus. One or two doses only.

*Sepia 30 or 200:* Weak, dragging or bearing down sensation in the uterus. Patient is tired and irritable. One or two doses.

### AROMATHERAPY
A course of tonifying massage after a miscarriage will help the body to recover more quickly. Consult an experienced aromatherapist.

For essential oils that should be avoided during pregnancy see PREGNANCY.

### BACH FLOWER REMEDIES
*Five Flower Remedy:* For fear, shock and anguish. Take a few drops as required.

For the emotional after effects of a miscarriage, or for fear of a miscarriage, consult the list in the Appendix, or look through a more detailed book on the Bach flower remedies and select the most appropriate remedies.


## MISCARRIAGE — ABORTION (AFTER EFFECTS)
A deliberately induced termination of pregnancy usually before sixteen weeks.

The following remedies may bring relief from some of the possible after effects of an abortion but consideration should be given to the need for ongoing emotional support and possible counselling. Be cautious about the possibility of any infection following an abortion: if suspected, seek urgent medical attention.

### HERBS
*Agnus Castus, Blue Cohosh, Chinese Angelica, Raspberry Leaf:* A tea to balance hormones and retone the uterus. Combine the herbs and make a decoction using one tea-

spoon of herbs to a mugful of water and simmer for ten minutes. Strain and drink a cupful three times a day, or use the tinctures, for two weeks.

*Skullcap, Valerian:* These may be added to the above mixture if there is a considerable amount of stress involved.

## HOMŒOPATHY

*Arnica 200:* For shock and bruising. Will also help to prevent haemorrhage and infection. Take one dose before the abortion and one dose afterwards.

*Bellis Perennis 30:* For the after effects of mechanical interference in the uterus. Bruised sensation in the abdomen. Yellow discharge. Two or three doses eight hours apart.

*Ignatia 200:* Grief and sadness dating from an abortion. One dose only.

*Staphysagria 200:* For after effects of mechanical interference in the womb, combined with unexpressed sadness and anger. One dose only.

## AROMATHERAPY

*Lavender:* Add five drops to the warm water for a soothing and healing bath.

*Neroli, Rose:* Uplifting and tonifying oils. Use for massage or in the bath.

## BACH FLOWER REMEDIES

*Five Flower Remedy:* For anguish, fear and shock. Take a few drops as often as required.

Look at the brief list in the Appendix of this book or study a more detailed book on the Bach flower remedies to help in selecting other appropriate remedies.


# MORNING SICKNESS

Symptoms include nausea, occasional vomiting and weakness. Some morning sickness is experienced by most women during the first few months of pregnancy. It is most frequently experienced in the morning, when the stomach is empty, although it may occur at any time of day. The traditional cure of eating a dry biscuit before rising is well worth trying. It seems to be caused by the massive upheaval of hormones occurring in the body, combined with low blood sugar. Symptoms usually recede after the third month of pregnancy, in which case professional help should be sought. Guidance should also be sought if vomiting is persistent, or any aversion to eating is prolonged.

Whilst it is best to avoid any medication during pregnancy, (unless specifically advised by your practitioner), the following remedies are gentle and safe and may help with this annoying symptom. Do consult your practitioner first if you are under treatment.

### HERBS

*Balm, Ginger (half), Meadowsweet:* This is a calming and soothing tea to help with nausea and acidity. Combine half quantity of *Ginger* to equal parts of the other herbs and infuse or take as tinctures three times a day.

### HOMŒOPATHY

*Ipecac 6 or30:* Persistent nausea that is not alleviated by vomiting. One or two doses daily as required.

*Nat Phos 6X:* Nausea with sour risings. One or two doses as required.

*Nux Vomica 6 or 30:* Nausea which is ameliorated by vomiting. Sour eructations, retching, indigestion. One or two doses as required.

*Pulsatilla 6 or 30:* Nausea with little vomiting and improved by fresh air. One or two doses as required.

*Sepia 6 or 30:* Nausea aggravated by the smell or thought of food, although it may be ameliorated by eating. Weak, sinking sensation in stomach. Vomiting. One or two doses as required.

## AROMATHERAPY

*Lavender:* One drop in a warm bath, or as a warm compress applied to the abdomen. (Warm a flannel in warm water and a drop of the oil. Place on the abdomen, wrap a large towel around you to keep warm.)

*Ginger, Peppermint:* Choose one of these and add a couple of drops to a tissue to inhale the vapours, or use in an essential oil burner.

# MOUTH ULCERS

Painful, small blisters on gums, tongue or mouth linings which are surrounded by redness. The appearance of mouth ulcers may indicate general debility. We recommend that care is taken with diet and rest, see CONVALESCENCE. If they occur regularly, seek constitutional treatment.

## HERBS

*Marigold, Myrrh, Red Sage, Thyme.* Mouth washes with any of the above herbs can be used either in the form of an infusion, or tinctures diluted in warm water.

## HOMŒOPATHY

*Borax 6 or 30:* Painful ulcers. Ulcers may bleed when touched. Aggravated by eating. One three times a day for up to five days.

*Mercurius 6 or 30:* Ulcers behind the tongue. Increased salivation. Metallic taste in mouth. Pain aggravated by heat and cold.One morning and night for up to five days.

*Nat Phos 6X:* Ulcers with acidic symptoms present. Sores and blisters on the tip of the tongue. One three times a day for five days.

## AROMATHERAPY

*Lavender, Myrrh, Tea Tree:* Dilute a couple of drops of one of these antiseptic and healing oils in a little alcohol (vodka) and water and use as a mouthwash.

## MUMPS

This is a highly infectious virus affecting the glands, usually the parotids, where swelling and tenderness will be noticed on the jawline. The first symptoms are often a mild fever and sore throat. Either one or both sides will be affected.

It is one of the common childhood diseases, and provides an opportunity to throw off inherited or acquired miasmatic influences. In children it is usually quite mild, but if occurring in adults, it may cause complications affecting the testicles in men and the ovaries in women. Although this rarely occurs, professional advice should be sought. Bed rest and plenty of fluids are recommended.

HERBS

*Balm, Cleavers, Echinacea, Yarrow:* Use equal quantities to make a soothing infusion which will also gently cleanse the glandular system. Drink a cupful three times a day. May be sweetened with honey.

HOMŒOPATHY

*Aconite 30:* Every six hours for first couple of days. First onset of symptoms — thirst, painful throat and fever.

*Apis 30:* One or two doses. Throat sore, swollen, painful, puffiness. Sharp or stinging pains. No thirst.

*Belladonna 30:* Two or three doses as necessary. Restless, burning. Swallowing difficult, high fever, light sensitive, throbbing pains.

*Clematis 30:* Swelling of glands under the jaw with throbbing pain, aggravated by touch. Painful swelling of testes. Two or three doses.

*Merc Sol 30:* Swelling of glands under jaw. Stitching pains to the ear on swallowing. Offensive odour from mouth; saliva increased. Feverish, thirsty. Two or three doses.

*Pulsatilla 30:* Swelling of glands under lower jaw or going to the testes. Bad taste in mouth. Child feels miserable and weepy, wants attention. Thirstless. Two or three doses.

AROMATHERAPY

*Roman Chamomile, Lavender:* Dilute a few drops of each in water and apply as a soothing and healing compress.

*Eucalyptus, Thyme:* Add a few drops of each to hot water for a steam inhalation that will be decongestant and assist the body to fight infection. These oils may also be sprayed in the patient's room.

# N

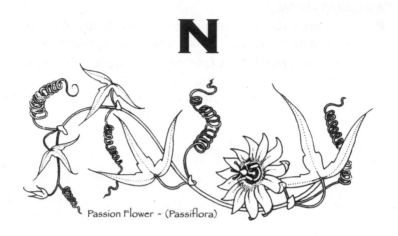

Passion Flower ~ (Passiflora)

## NAUSEA

This can vary from a slight feeling of queasiness to an overwhelming urge to vomit. Causes of nausea can be either psychological or physiological. Refer to the appropriate cross-reference or, if nausea is persistent, seek diagnosis from a practitioner. Any form of dietary indiscretion could result in nausea. The following remedies will help with an occasional bout of nausea.

(See also: ALLERGY, ANXIETY, GASTROENTERITIS, HANGOVER, INDIGESTION, MIGRAINE, MORNING SICKNESS, STRESS, SUNSTROKE.)

### HERBS

*Balm, Chamomile, Ginger, Meadowsweet, Peppermint, Vervain:* An infusion of any of these herbs singly or as a combination will bring soothing relief to feelings of nausea.

*Cardamon Seeds:* If nausea results from eating a heavy meal, chewing a few of these seeds will bring quick amelioration.

### HOMŒOPATHY

*Ipecac 6 or 30:* Horrid nausea not relieved by vomiting. Thirstless. Sinking sensation in the stomach. Clean tongue. One dose every few hours.

*Kali Mur 6X:* Nausea after eating rich or fatty foods. The tongue has a white or greyish coating. One dose every three to four hours.

*Kali Phos 6X:* Nausea caused by nervousness. 'All gone' sensation in the stomach. One dose every three to four hours.

*Nat Phos 6X:* Nausea with sour risings. Brought on after eating fruit or acid food. Yellow coating to tongue. One dose every three to four hours.

*Nat Sulph 6X:* Nausea with bilious symptoms. Brought on after eating fatty food. Bitter taste in the mouth. Greenish coating to tongue. One dose every three to four hours.

*Nux Vom 6 or 30:* Nausea brought on from over-indulgence in food or alcohol. Nausea relieved by vomiting. Feels irritable. One dose every few hours.

AROMATHERAPY

*Cardamom, Fennel, Ginger, Melissa, Peppermint:* A few drops of either of these oils in a little vegetable oil and massaged into the stomach area will relieve feelings of nausea.


## NEURALGIA

Neuralgia is a painful condition originating from an inflamed nerve. The most common sites are the trigeminal nerves in the face, and the sciatic nerve which causes pain in the lower back and thighs. A fortifying diet with particular attention to additional B complex vitamins will help this condition.

HERBS

*Oats, Passiflora, St John's Wort, Skullcap:* These herbs are anti-inflammatory and soothing to the nerves. Combine and make an infusion using one teaspoon per cup, drink three cupfuls a day.

HOMŒOPATHY

*Calc Phos 6X:* Use afterwards as a nerve restorative. Morning and night for ten days.

*Ferrum Phos 6X:* Acute neuralgic pains due to inflammation, caused by chills, fever, etc. One dose three times a day.

*Hypericum 30:* Tingling, burning and numbness, worse after injury, or caused by injury. Very severe nerve pain. One dose three times a day for five days.

*Kali Phos 6X:* A nerve nutrient, restlessness, exhaustion and neuralgic pain. May be taken in alternation with *Mag Phos*. Two doses a day for ten days.

*Mag Phos 6X:* Shooting, spasmodic neuralgic pains aggravated by cold. Alternate with *Kali Phos*. Two doses daily for ten days.

*Spigelia 30:* Trigeminal neuralgia with violent burning and stitching pains radiating outwards. Worse for touch. One dose a day for three days.

AROMATHERAPY

*Chamomile, Lavender, Marjoram, Rosemary:* Add to *St John's Wort* macerated oil or other vegetable base oil for a local massage or compress. Also combine, or use separately, and add to a base bath oil before adding to a warm bath as often as required.

# NOSEBLEEDS

This may occur as a result of injury to the nose, or sometimes from disorders of the blood. If the delicate veins inside the nose are damaged by a previous accident, then even a trivial knock to the area will trigger off a nosebleed.

In children, nosebleeds are very common. If an adult suddenly develops recurring nosebleeds, then professional advice should be sought.

A course of bioflavonoid *(Rutin)* tablets will help

strengthen the vein walls if nosebleeds are frequent. First-aid measures include pinching the nose or placing an ice-cold compress on the back of the neck for a few minutes until the bleeding ceases.

## HERBS
*St Johns Wort, Witchazel, Yarrow:* These are astringents to encourage the bleeding to stop. Make an infusion to saturate a piece of cotton wool and hold under the nose.

## HOMŒOPATHY
*Aconite 30:* Nosebleed triggered by a shock or fright. One or two doses.

*Arnica 30:* Nosebleed after injury or trauma to the nose. Nosebleed after a fit of coughing. One or two doses.

*Ferrum Phos 6X:* Bright red blood. Nosebleeds in children. One or two doses.

*Phosphorus 30:* Nosebleeds in nervous types. Bright blood slow to stop. One or two doses.

## AROMATHERAPY
*Cypress, Yarrow:* A few drops of essential oil applied to cotton wool and held under the nose for a few moments will arrest bleeding.

# O

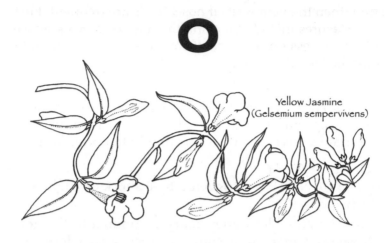

Yellow Jasmine
(Gelsemium sempervivens)

## OBESITY

A condition arising from excess of fat, generally brought about by overeating, or eating the wrong foods. Often psychological or cultural factors determine our opinions on what is a fat person and what isn't. We feel that the correct weight for a person is very individual; based on the optimum efficiency of the body. This is creating a balance between two opposites — a weakness brought about by being underweight, and sluggishness and other problems arising from fatness.

Too many carbohydrates alongside insufficient exercise produces fat which stays in the body. Fat people run a greater risk of ill-health, including heart and circulation problems and diseases of the kidneys.

Reducing fat in the body can really only be brought about naturally by eating less carbohydrates and increasing the output of energy. Slimming, or rather weight reduction, requires common sense in both psychological and nutritional terms. Counselling alongside diet control is advisable. Evidence suggests that a balanced wholefood diet is preferable; consult a naturopath or other natural physicians for advice.

## HERBS

*Bladderwrack:* A nourishing sea plant that stimulates the metabolism and may help obesity when taken in conjunction with an appropriate diet. Drink the infusion or take the tincture or capsules three times a day for several weeks.

# OPERATIONS
# (PREPARATION AND AFTER EFFECTS)

Post-operational distress and depression can be somewhat alleviated by supplementing the diet with vitamin B. It is recommended that people taking garlic supplements should cease 10 days before surgery due to its antiplatelet activity.

## HERBS

*Calendula, Comfrey, St John's Wort:* These will promote healing and help to reduce scarring. Make an infusion to bathe the affected area or apply as an ointment.

## HOMŒOPATHY

*Arnica 200:* One dose before and one dose daily for a few days after the operation to help with shock and promote rapid healing.

*Calendula 30:* Promotes healing of the skin and tissues after surgery. Helps prevent scarring. One dose twice a day for one week.

*Hypericum 30:* Promotes healing of any nerve damage and relieves the pain of surgery to areas rich in nerves. Also helps prevent infection. One dose twice a day for one week.

*Phosphorus 30:* For nausea and exhaustion following an anaesthetic. One or two doses.

## AROMATHERAPHY

*Lavender, Helichrysum, Patchouli, Rose:* Add a few drops of each oil to a vegetable oil base to promote healing and reduce scarring. Gently massage in on and around the affected area.

## BACH FLOWER REMEDIES

*Five Flower Remedy*: Take whenever necessary before and after; for anticipation, shock and trauma.

# P

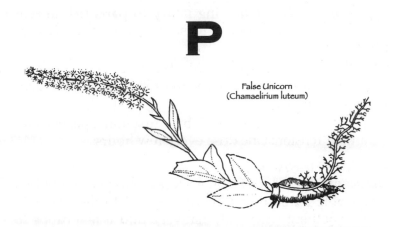

False Unicorn
(Chamaelirium luteum)

## PAIN

This is not an illness in itself, but a reaction to a physical or psychological cause, and it is that cause which one needs to identify and treat (getting rid of the sensation of pain without treating the cause can be beneficial in the short term, but it is often counter-productive in the long term).

An individual's response to pain varies from time to time as well as from person to person, and thus pains without a direct physiological cause should be referred to a holistic therapist. Those suffering from chronic pain also should seek advice. Obviously, acute pain should be treated according to its specific cause, but the following remedies may offer general help for pain-relief in the short term.

### HERBS

*Skullcap, Valerian, White Willow:* All these have a mild pain relieving effect. Combine, infuse and drink a cupful every few hours.

### HOMŒOPATHY

*Arnica 30:* Pain resulting from an injury or blow. Two or three doses.

*Ferrum Phos 6X:* Pain due to inflammation. Heat and redness may be present. One dose every few hours.

131

*Hypericum 30:* Pain following injury to parts rich in sentient nerves, e.g., fingers, toes, or to the spine. Two or three doses.

*Kali Phos 6X:* For pain involving nerve endings. Aggravated by nervousness and exhaustion. One dose every few hours.

*Mag Phos 6X:* Pains caused by muscular spasms and cramps. Tension. One dose every few hours.

## AROMATHERAPY
*Chamomile, Lavender, Marjoram:* A few drops of these in a vegetable oil base and gently applied to the area will offer soothing relief. Alternatively, add a few drops to the bath.

## BACH FLOWER REMEDIES
*Five Flower Remedy:* Take internally as drops or apply externally onto the affected area.

*Five Flower Cream:* Apply to the affected area.

# PANIC ATTACKS
See: ANXIETY

# PILL (AFTER EFFECTS)
The advent of the contraceptive pill has enabled women to have greater sexual freedom, but at a loss. Although information on the side-effects of the pill has been available, it is often not taken seriously enough. Basically, the pill controls the hormonal system and, therefore, subtley controls the emotional side of the woman. The pill can be contributory in causing heart disease, thrombosis, cervical cancer, vaginal infections, weight gain and nausea.

When you stop taking the pill, the following remedies may assist in re-adjusting the hormonal balance of the body. If any problems persist, or you suspect you may be pregnant, consult a practitioner.

HERBS

*Agnus Castus, Black Cohosh, Chinese Angelica:* A mixture to assist in the functioning of the ovaries and re-balancing the hormones. Combine equal quantities, decoct or use the tinctures and drink twice daily for four to five weeks. If you suspect you may be pregnant, do not take the herbs, but consult professional advice.

## PALPITATIONS

Palpitations are caused either by the heart beating more forcibly, or the person's increased awareness of the heart beat. They are often transient and harmless and pass once the sufferer is able to relax. However, more prolonged episodes of palpitations, with rapid pulse, will need urgent medical assessment as this may indicate an underlying heart problem. Be cautious: if there is any departure from a previously stable pattern, seek medical advice, as an electrocardiogram can often provide a clear cut diagnosis.

The following remedies will offer relief in cases of mild palpitations where there is an obvious cause, such as nervous tension, and no other symptoms of heart trouble, e.g. chest tightness, dizziness, shortness of breath.

HERBS

*Balm, Hawthorn, Lime Flowers, Motherwort, Passiflora:* Combine the herbs and make an infusion using one heaped teaspoon of herbs to one cupful of boiling water, stand for ten minutes before straining. Alternatively use the tinctures. This may be taken three times a day.

HOMŒOPATHY

*Aconite 30:* Palpitations due to fright or shock. Fears may die any minute. Panic attacks.

*Kali Phos 6X:* Nervous palpitations. One dose every few hours as required.

AROMATHERAPY
*Melissa, Neroli, Ylang Ylang:* Add one or two drops of either of the oils to a warm bath, or add a few drops of each to a little vegetable oil base to use as a massage oil.

## PERIOD PAINS
(See: MENSTRUAL PROBLEMS)

## PLEURISY
Inflammation of the pleural membranes which surround the lungs. Pleurisy is often a secondary complaint associated with other lung diseases. The symptoms are pain on coughing, and when drawing in air. It may be accompanied with a fever.

Professional medical advice is essential when dealing with this complaint.

(See also: BRONCHITIS, CONVALESCENCE.)

## PNEUMONIA
Inflammation of the lungs. This can occur on its own or as a secondary complaint of other illnesses.

Any sudden or long-term fever associated with a cough, especially with blood-tinged sputum, should arouse the suspicion of possible pneumonia. Immediate medical advice must be sought.

(See also: BRONCHITIS, CONVALESCENCE.)

## POST-NATAL DEPRESSION
Most women will feel exhausted immediately after giving birth, and with successive disturbed nights, and the hormonal changes occurring at this time, re-adjustment to the new life with a baby can be worrying. Some women will experience actual depression after giving birth. If this becomes severe, or continues for more than a day or two,

seek immediate professional advice. The following remedies will supplement professional help and relieve mild feelings of depression or post-natal blues.
(See also: CONVALESCENCE.)

## HERBS
*Agnus Castus, Balm, Oat, Squaw Vine, Vervain:* A useful tonic to balance the hormones and nervous system. Take as tinctures or make an infusion and drink each morning and evening.

## HOMŒOPATHY
Seek constitutional treatment according to individual symptoms.

## AROMATHERAPY
*Clary Sage, Geranium, Jasmine, Melissa, Neroli:* Combine two or three of the oils, or use separately, adding either to a bath oil, or in a massage base oil, and use regularly.

## BACH FLOWER REMEDIES
Study the Bach flower literature (see Appendix) or consult an experienced practitioner to find the appropriate remedy. *Cherry Plum, Mustard, Olive, Willow* may be worth special consideration.

# PREGNANCY
Whilst pregnancy is, of course, a completely natural process, it can place a lot of demands upon the emotions and body of a woman. Generally speaking, if you are feeling well, then it is better not to interfere in any way with the natural processes occuring at this time; but having said that, there is growing pressure on women today to keep active, and also have an entirely healthy and natural pregnancy and labour, which can feel quite overwhelming. Alternative medicine has many useful and safe treatments to assist a woman during this time, and the suggestions that follow will offer aid for certain problems; but ideally, a pregnant woman would benefit most

from constitutional and specific treatment that could be offered by a qualified natural therapist.

Of course, where possible, any drug medication should be avoided, as should stimulants, alcohol and cigarettes. There are many herbs and essential oils that, whilst perfectly safe to use at other times, may have an abortifacient effect and should be avoided during pregnancy. The following list comprises of those common herbs and oils which should not be used during pregnancy.

(See also: ANÆMIA, BREAST-FEEDING, CONST-IPATION, GASTRITIS, INDIGESTION, INSOMNIA, LABOUR, MORNING SICKNESS, POST-NATAL DEPRESSION, STRETCH MARKS, VARICOSE VEINS.)

## HERBS TO AVOID DURING PREGNANCY

*Aloes, Angelica, Barberry, Bethroot, Black Cohosh, Bloodroot, Blue Cohosh, Buckthorn, Cascara Sagrada, Catnip, Celery Seed, Cinchona, Coltsfoot, Cottonroot, Elecampane, Fenugreek, Feverfew, Ginseng, Gotu kola, Goldenseal, Greater Celandine, Holy Thistle, Hops, Horsetail, Hyssop, Juniper, Lady's Mantle, Liferoot, Liquorice, Male Fern, Mandrake, Marigold, Milk Thistle, Motherwort, Myrrh, Pennyroyal, Pokeroot, Prickly Ash, Red Clover, Rhubarb, Rosemary, Rue, Saffron, Sage, Senna, Shepherd's Purse, Southernwood, Tansy, Thuja, Uva Ursi, Vervain, White Horehound, Wild Indigo, Wild Yam, Wormwood, Yarrow, Yellow Dock.*

These herbs should not be taken internally in therapeutic doses during pregnancy. Culinary doses are acceptable. Generally speaking, the list includes those herbs acting as abortifacients, emmenagogues and strong laxatives. Really, any herb taken in therapeutic dosage should be specifically checked for use during pregnancy.

---

# ESSENTIAL OILS TO AVOID
# DURING PREGNANCY
*Basil, Camphor, Hyssop, Pennyroyal, Sage, Savoury, Thuja, Wintergreen.*

---

## HERBS

### PREPARATION FOR LABOUR

*Raspberry leaf:* This tea drunk on a regular basis through-out the last three months of pregnancy will strengthen the uterine and pelvic muscles and help to make the birth easier. One heaped teaspoon to a cup of boiling water and infuse for ten minutes. Drink two or three times a day.

*Squaw Vine:* Drink regularly during the last two months of pregnancy to prepare the uterus for birth. One tea-spoonful per cup of boiling water, drink a cupful daily. May be combined with Raspberry leaves.

### AFTER-BIRTH BATH

*Comfrey, Marigold, St Johns Wort, Shepherd's Purse:* Combine the above herbs and make into an infusion using one tablespoon to a pint of boiling water. After ten minutes strain, and pour the infusion into a bath of warm water and sit in the bath water for a soothing and healing bath. Alternatively, use the infusion, when cool, externally by applying to the perineum with cotton wool.

### HEALING

*Calendula and Hypericum Tincture:* Add a few drops of the tinctures to a small bowl of warm water. Apply with cotton wool to heal tears or stitches.

## HOMŒOPATHY

*Calc Fluor 6X:* Gives elasticity to tissues, so helps prevent stretch marks and tones up the pelvic area. Also useful for the formation of healthy teeth and bones in the foetus. Take one dose twice a day for ten days at any time during pregnancy.

*Ferrum Phos 6X:* An alternative to synthetic iron tablets. Encourages the body to assimilate iron more effectively. One dose two times a day for up to one month.

## AROMATHERAPY

*Frankincense (Olibanum), Mandarin, Neroli:* A few drops of these oils in a vegetable base oil may be used for a pleasant, soothing massage at any time during pregnancy. They will also help to prevent stretch marks.

*Wheatgerm Oil:* This oil is rich in vitamin E and will help prevent stretch marks. It is a heavy oil and thus will be easier to use if combined with a lighter oil such as *Almond* or *Apricot Kernel* oil. Massage into the skin regularly.

## GENERAL SUPPLEMENTS

It can be necessary to increase the intake of iron during pregnancy. Rather than taking synthetic iron tablets which may cause indigestion or constipation, we suggest either: *Nettle* tea; *Ferrum Phos* (see Homœopathy); or Floradix — a herbally based iron-rich tonic available from health food shops.

# PRE-MENSTRUAL TENSION

Hormonal changes are occurring all the time in women of menstruating age, and the individual's response will vary according to the constitution and general well-being of the body and emotions.

Physical symptoms frequently experienced by many women pre-menstrually include: nausea, headaches, bloatedness, swollen breasts, spots and other skin changes (see the relevant headings in the book).

Increasing acceptance in our society of Pre-Menstrual Tension (PMT) may allow women to express and justify otherwise unacceptable emotions that are accentuated during these cyclic changes. Women that suffer distressing emotional symptoms prior to their periods could take this as an opportunity not to suppress these feelings, but to look at their general well-being in our stress-filled society; maybe with the help of a professional therapist. As with so many problems, alleviating PMT is usually a process that will include several lifestyle factors. In particular, the symptoms of congestion and irritability may benefit from going on a cleansing diet combined with remedies to balance the hormones.

Whilst we recognise that there is an inter-relationship between emotional and physical symptoms which should be explored for any condition, the following suggestions will help with the most commonly experienced physical symptoms that occur pre-menstrually; mainly due to salt and water accumulating in the tissues as a response to the hormonal secretions preceding menstruation.

(See also: MENSTRUAL PROBLEMS.)

## HERBS

*Agnus Castus, Chinese Angelica:* These herbs have the effect of stabilising the hormones. Combine and make a decoction to drink three times a day as a course of treatment for up to three months. Alternatively take as tinctures.

*Motherwort, Passiflora, Scullcap:* Drink a combination of these herbs as an infusion or tinctures three times a day when there are symptoms of anxiety and stress present.

*Cramp Bark:* This may be taken if there are cramping pains present.

*Dandelion Leaves:* An infusion drunk three times a day can be used as a diuretic to ease bloatedness and other symptoms of water retention.

## HOMŒOPATHY

There are homœopathic remedies to help deal with these distressing symptoms, but one must consult a homœopath for individual treatment to obtain full benefit.

## AROMATHERAPY

*Clary Sage, Geranium, Rose:* Any of these oils used as a few drops in the bath or in a massage oil will soothe symptoms of stress and discomfort.

*Juniper:* A few drops diluted in vegetable oil and massaged in, or added to a bath, will have a diuretic effect.

## BACH FLOWER REMEDIES

These will undoubtedly be of assistance by working on the emotional causes of PMT. We suggest you refer to the appropriate literature, and choose the remedies most suitable for your needs.

## GENERAL

*Evening Primrose Oil:* Either in capsule form, or taken as the oil itself, has proved to be of great benefit to some sufferers of the symptoms of PMT. As a guide to dosage, we suggest 1 x 500 mg per day for the first month, and then 1 x 500 mg per day for the appropriate ten days preceeding menstruation for succeeding months. This works especially well for painful or swollen breasts.

Similarly, many people have obtained benefit from vitamin therapy, in particular B6.

# PSORIASIS

Over-production of skin cells usually presenting itself on bony areas of the body, e.g. shins, elbows or scalp. Symptoms include flaking of the skin, often accompanied by itching.

There is a hereditary factor to this disease, although it will also be aggravated by stress or trauma. Symptoms are often alleviated by sunshine and sea bathing. *Evening Primrose Oil* or *Flax Seed Oil* may also be of benefit. Constitutional treatment is definitely recommended to get to the root of this disease.

## HERBS

A qualified herbalist should be consulted for effective treatment, but the following herbs may assist.

*Blue Flag Root, Burdock Root, Red Clover, Sarsaparilla, Yellow Dock:* A combination of these herbs may be taken as a decoction or as tinctures three times daily over a period of time, up to three months.

## HOMŒOPATHY

Consult a qualified practitioner.

## AROMATHERAPY

*Bergamot, Cedarwood, Helichrysum, Lavender, Sandalwood:* Choose two or three of these oils to add to a vegetable oil base and massage into affected areas daily.

# R

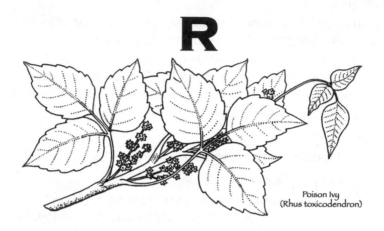

Poison Ivy
(Rhus toxicodendron)

## RHEUMATISM

Inflammation of the connective tissues covering the muscles, and of the tendons, also known as myalgia, fibrositis and lumbago. The muscles in the area of the inflammation tighten as a defensive reaction and when this happens the nearby joint may become deformed. Hence, rheumatism and arthritis may often become confused.

Rheumatic fever is an acute form of rheumatism found mostly in children, heralded by sore throat and followed one to three weeks later by fever with transient joint pains, and occasionally muscular spasms. It should be treated by a qualified practitioner, due to the risk of inflammatory damage to the heart.

The treatment of rheumatism is similar to that of arthritis, and both are the result of an inappropriate diet which reduces the body's ability to eliminate toxic waste matter, combined with stress and tension in the lifestyle having its counterpart in the body, and a hereditary factor. Whilst the following suggestions will offer some alleviation from the discomfort of rheumatism, a holistic approach involving advice on diet, exercise and lifestyle is necessary to cure the problem. Constitutional treatment by a qualified holistic practitioner is recommended.

(See also: ARTHRITIS.)

## HERBS

### INTERNAL

*Bogbean:* If the condition is aggravated in damp weather, add this to the following mixture.

*Celery Seed, Dandelion, Meadowsweet, Nettle, White Willow:* A combination of these herbs will encourage the body to eliminate toxins and help with pain and inflammation.

*Devil's Claw:* This is a popular remedy for rheumatism. Soak a couple of pieces of the root in two cupfuls of water. The following morning boil up the root and water for ten to fifteen minutes, and then drink the liquid. Repeat daily.

### EXTERNAL

*Comfrey Oil:* Massage this oil over the affected area.

*Rhus Tox Ointment:* Rub into affected area.

## HOMŒOPATHY

*Arnica 30:* Limbs ache as if beaten, affected parts feel sore and bruised. Rheumatic pains brought on by injury or over-exertion. One dose two times daily for up to ten days.

*Bryonia 30:* Heaviness of the limbs with redness and swelling of the joints. Patient feels compelled to keep the affected part still. Irritability. One dose twice daily for up to ten days.

*Ferrum Phos 6X:* Acute attacks of rheumatism. For pain, inflammation and congestion. One dose three times daily for up to ten days.

*Nat Phos 6X:* The acid neutralising tissue salt. Breaks up the harmful acids. One dose three times daily for up to ten days. May be taken in conjunction with Nat Sulph.

*Nat Sulph 6X:* Encourages removal of toxic charged fluids from the system. One dose three times daily for up to ten days.

*Rhus Tox 30:* Swelling and stiffness of limbs brought on by over-lifting or over-stretching. Also worse in cold, damp weather. Better from gentle motion, stiffens up during rest. One dose three times daily for up to ten days.

AROMATHERAPY

*Juniper, Pine:* A few drops of either of these oils in a bowl of warm water and use as a local bath or compress.

*Benzoin, Eucalyptus, Lavender, Marjoram, Rosemary:* Add a few drops of each oil to *Comfrey* macerated oil or any vegetable base oil and massage into the area.


## RINGWORM

A fungal infection of the skin which occurs on various parts of the body. The infection tends to spread outwards in a disc, the centre heals while the circumference is still active and forms a reddish circle. Scrupulous hygiene will be necessary to eliminate this problem as well as local healing applications. If the condition persists, constitutional treatment by a qualified therapist will be necessary.

HERBS

*Echinacea, Marigold, Myrrh:* Combine tinctures of the above and apply locally to the area.

AROMATHERAPY

*Myrrh, Tea Tree:* Apply either of these, undiluted, to the affected area.

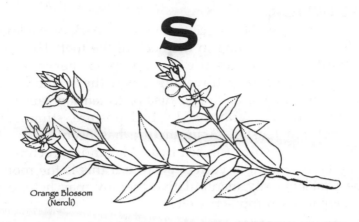

Orange Blossom
(Neroli)

## SCABIES

A skin disease caused by a tiny parasitic insect which burrows under the skin, normally in the soft fleshy parts of the body, and never above the neck line. Scrupulous hygiene is imperative to prevent spreading. Before using orthodox treatment, some of the following could be tried:

### HERBS

*Quassia, Tansy:* A strong decoction should be made using 25 g of each herb to a pint and applied to the whole body twice a day.

### HOMŒOPATHY

*Staphisagria 30:* One dose a day for five days in conjunction with external applications. Crawling sensation on the skin.

*Sulphur 6:* To improve quality of skin and help with itching, one dose morning and night for ten days.

### AROMATHERAPY

*Bergamot, Cedarwood, Clove, Eucalyptus, Rosemary, Tea Tree:* Combine a few drops of each in a vegetable oil base and apply to affected areas.

## SCIATICA

Pain in the area of the sciatic nerve i.e. back of the knee, calf or even extending to the back of the foot. The commonest cause is pressure on the spinal nerve which causes referred pain travelling down the sciatic nerve. Sometimes due to a slipped disc or to tension causing a trapped nerve aggravated by bad posture, stimulants, alcohol and tension. Acupuncture has been known to have good results for sciatica. Alexander Technique may be beneficial to correct posture if this is the root of the problem. Any manipulative therapy may help, e.g., Osteopathy, Chiropractice etc.

Prolonged episodes may result in damage to the sciatic nerve so careful treatment by an experienced practitioner is vital.

(See also: NEURALGIA.)

## SHINGLES (HERPES ZOSTER)

Shingles is caused by a virus, similar to that which causes chicken pox. The distinguishing symptom is of painful clusters of blisters at the nerve endings. The patient feels generally unwell, and may be feverish during the acute attack. The pain may persist even when the blisters have gone.

An attack of shingles is often an indication of general debility and patients should have an improved diet and plenty of rest. Extra vitamins, and especially eating more foods rich in B vitamins will help.

The advice that follows applies to shingles on the chest, buttocks, etc.; shingles on the forehead or anywhere near the eyes should be treated only under the supervision of a medical practitioner.

## HERBS

INTERNAL

*Oats, Skullcap, St John's Wort, Vervain:* Combine these nervine relaxants and tonics and make an infusion using a heaped teaspoon of dried herbs to a cupful of boiling water or use the tinctures. Take three times a day.

EXTERNAL

*St John's Wort:* Apply the macerated oil to the affected areas to bring relief and promote healing.

## HOMŒOPATHY

*Ars Alb 6 or 30:* Intense burning, with relief from warmth. Anxious and restless patient. One 30th potency a day for three days or one 6th potency three times a day for up to ten days.

*Kali Phos 6X:* Lightning pains along the nerves. A nerve nutrient useful to take after the initial attack. One dose three times a day for ten days.

*Mezereum 6 or 30:* Intolerable itching and painful eruptions aggravated by warmth and when in bed. Pain remains after the eruptions have gone. One 30th potency a day for three days or one 6th potency three times a day for up to ten days.

*Rhus Tox 6 or 30:* Intense itching with painful, watery blisters. Blisters on parts of the body covered with hair. One 30th potency a day for three days or one 6th potency three times a day for up to ten days.

## AROMATHERAPY

*Lavender, Ravensasra:* Make a strong dilution in *St John's Wort* macerated oil or other vegetable base oil to apply directly onto the affected areas.

## SHOCK

Technically shock is a reaction that occurs when the blood flow is reduced below the levels necessary to supply oxygen to the nervous system. Some degree of shock can occur after any injury, burn or illness that involves loss of blood or other body fluids. It can also occur during infection, allergic reaction or malfunction of the nervous system.

Symptoms of shock are: general weakness, cold, clammy, pale skin, a rapid, weak pulse, reduced alertness and shallow, irregular breathing. Nausea may also be present. Hot sweetened tea would help for minor shock.

One should suspect shock with any injury, and apply first-aid measures, whilst, if the injury appears severe, calling emergency aid. Reassure the patient, and get them to lay down with their feet slightly raised above the level of dieir head (except in the case of a head or chest injury where the head should be higher than the feet).

The following remedies will help for minor cases of shock, or may be administered whilst awaiting emergency medical treatment in more severe cases.

(See also: ACCIDENTS.)

### HERBS

*Balm, Chamomile, Peppermint, Skullcap:* Make an infusion and sweeten with honey to drink when required.

### HOMŒOPATHY

*Aconite 30:* Shock with extreme fear and panic. Nightmares following shock. Two or three doses.

*Arnica 30 or 200:* Shock from an accident or physical injury. Two or three doses.

*Chamomilla 30:* Shock where the patient is hysterical with the pain. Two or three doses.

*China 30:* Shock from loss of blood or other vital fluids. Two or three doses.

*Ignatia 30:* Shock from grief or fright with hysteria and fainting. Two or three doses.

## AROMATHERAPY

*Lavender, Melissa, Neroli, Peppermint:* Use whichever is available. Hold under the patient's nose. Could also be used in a massage oil for delayed or emotional shock.

## BACH FLOWER REMEDIES

*Five Flower Remedy:* An invaluable aid at the time of shock. Take a few drops frequently, undiluted if necessary.

# SINUSITIS

Infection or inflammation of the sinus cavities which often leads to increased mucous production. Symptoms include pain at the root of the nose, above or below the eyes, and a sensation of stuffiness in the head. Acute sinusitis may be accompanied by a fever and severe headache. It can become chronic and is often aggravated by colds, hayfever, emotional upset or damp weather. This should be treated constitutionally by a qualified practitioner. Acute attacks can often be managed by self-care, but any deterioration in the patient's condition is a signal for seeking medical advice.

We recommend a dairy-free diet to keep down mucus formation, and *Garlic* capsules to prevent infection.

## HERBS

*Echinacea, ElderFlower, Eyebright, Golden Rod, Golden Seal (half), Marshmallow:* Combine and infuse or use the tinctures. This mixture drunk two times daily will help release blocked mucus and soothe inflammation.

## HOMŒOPATHY

*Bryonia 6 or 30:* Heavy frontal headache; dryness and pressure sensation in nose; irritable. One dose of the 6 potency three times a day for five days or one dose of 30 a day for three days.

*Kali Bich 6 or 30:* Pressure or stuffed-up sensation at root of nose. Thick, stringy, yellow discharge. Localised frontal headache, especially over eyebrows; very pain-ful. One 30 potency a day for three days, or one 6 three times a day for five days.

*Kali Sulph 6 or 30:* Nose bunged up; worse in warm room and evening; loss of taste; yellow catarrh. One 30 potency a day for three days or one 6 three times a day for five days.

*Merc Sol 6 or 30:* Infected catarrhal inflammation of frontal sinuses. Pain worse at night, purulent discharge, offen-sive taste in mouth. One 30 potency a day for three days or one 6 three times a day for five days.

*Spigelia 6 or 30:* Dryness of nose with post-nasal dripping. Neuralgic pains in cheeks or over eyes. One 30 potency a day for three days or one 6 three times a day for five days.

AROMATHERAPY
*Eucalyptus, Pine, Ravensara:* Use a few drops of one of these oils as a steam inhalation.


## SLEEPLESSNESS
(See: INSOMNIA.)


## SORE THROAT
This is often the first indication of the onset of an illness. Most sore throats are self-limiting and symptoms will go with rest, fresh fruit and vegetables and plenty to drink. The following remedies will offer relief for any unaccept-able discomfort. A simple soothing drink may be made from lemon juice and a teaspoon of honey in hot water. If symptoms persist or a high fever develops, call for pro-fessional advice.

(See also: COLDS, MUMPS, TONSILLITIS.)

HERBS
*Red Sage:* Make an infusion using a heaped teaspoon to a cup of boiling water, stand for ten minutes, strain and

use as a gargle. This may also be drunk as a soothing tea.

*Balm of Gilead, Echinacea, Elderberry:* If the sore throat drags on, this mixture will be soothing and encourage the body to throw off the symptoms. Make a decoction simmering a teaspoon of herbs to a cupful of boiling water for ten minutes or use the tinctures. Take three times a day.

## HOMŒOPATHY

*Aconite 30:* Sore throat preceding a cold or childhood illness. First stages. Two or three doses.

*Belladonna 30:* Sore throat and swollen, red tonsils. Fever with congested, red, hot face and skin. Take one dose of the 30th potency twice a day for three days.

*Ferrum Phos 6X:* Sore throat and hoarseness. Occurs when feeling run down. Redness and inflammation. One dose three times daily.

*Hepar Sulph 30:* Swelling of throat and glands in neck. Soreness. Sensation of fish bones in throat. Patient chilly and irritable. Take one dose of the 30th potency twice a day for three days.

*Lachesis 30:* Sensation of soreness and lump in the throat. Aggravated by swallowing. Pains move from left to right or are left-sided. Take one dose of the 30th potency twice a day for three days.

*Merc Sol 30:* Sore, raw throat, slow to improve. Feverishness worse at night. Swollen glands. Offensive breath. Painful swallowing. Take one dose of the 30th potency twice a day for three days.

## AROMATHERAPY

*Lemon, Niaouli, Thyme:* Add two drops of each oil to hot water and use as a steam inhalation.

## SPLINTERS

A foreign object beneath the skin. The object should be removed as quickly as possible to prevent infection.

### HERBS

*Hypericum and Calendula Ointment:* Put on a plaster to help draw out the splinter.

*Slippery Elm:* A warm poultice of the powder will help draw out the splinter..

### HOMŒOPATHY

*Hypericum 6 or 30:* If it is very painful. Take three doses of the 6th potency a day for five days, or one dose of the 30th potency a day for three days.

*Silica 6X:* To encourage the body to expel the splinter. One three times a day for two to three days.

### AROMATHERAPY

*Lavender, Tea Tree:* Apply neat over area to be treated and then put on a plaster to draw the splinter out.


## SPRAINS AND STRAINS

An injury that tears or stretches supporting tissue of a joint; usually of ankles, wrists, fists or knees. To take strain off the affected joint whilst it heals, a supporting bandage may be required.

Cold water compressess may offer immediate relief. If symptoms appear at all severe, be aware that it may be a fracture and seek medical help.

(See also: ACCIDENTS.)

### HERBS

*Arnica, Comfrey, Witchazel:* Use as tinctures or make an infusion for an external application — soak a cloth in the liquid and apply to the area as a compress.

OINTMENTS

*Arnica:* Immediately after the injury for bruising and pain. Do not use on broken skin.

*Rhus Tox:* Injury to muscles. Swelling, pain and stiffness.

*Ruta:* Injury to ligaments and tendons. Massage well into the joint to promote rapid healing.

HOMŒOPATHY

*Arnica 30:* Use immediately after the injury for shock and to promote healing. Two or three doses.

*Bellis Perennis30:* Muscles and joints sore and bruised. Swelling after an injury. After gardening. Three times a day for five days.

*Rhus Tox 30:* Sprains that are sore, stiff and swollen. Area becomes stiff during rest and ameliorated by continued gentle movement. Painful on first moving. Three times a day for five days.

*Ruta 30:* Injury to ligaments, tendons and cartilage. Painful joints. Three times a day for five days. May be taken in conjunction with Rhus tox.

*Black Pepper, Lavender, Rosemary:* Combine oils and use on a warm cloth as a compress, or add the oils to a bowl of warm water and bathe the affected part.

## STRESS

We seem to be able to adapt to a certain amount of stress in our lives without showing symptoms of disease, indeed some stress may even be considered necessary for growth and development, but at some point, if excess stress continues, or a new one is added, the balance is tipped and we begin to experience symptoms of one kind or another as a result.

The only way that we are going to be able to reduce the amount of stress in our lives is to choose another way of doing things; it may be that consulting with a practitioner is part of the process of reassessing and dealing with an unhealthy level of stress in our lives. The B vitamins are used up rapidly when we are experiencing stress and a B complex may be taken to help support the nervous system. The following remedies may help us whilst going through a particularly stressful phase, or whilst reassessing our lifestyle but should only be taken for a few weeks at a time along with sorting out the things that are causing our stress in the first place.

(See also: ANXIETY, INSOMNIA)

## HERBS

*Balm, Chamomile, Passiflora, Skullcap, Vervain:* An effective blend of herbs that will support our nervous system and relieve symptoms of stress such as sleeplessness and anxiety. Combine the herbs and make an infusion or use the tinctures and take three times a day when required.

*Siberian Ginseng:* An herb known as an adaptogen that increases the capacity of the body to cope with physical and mental stress. Take the tincture three times a day for several weeks.

## HOMŒOPATHY

*Calc Phos, Kali Phos, Mag Phos 6X:* Relieves symptoms of nervous fatigue, sleeplessness, stress headaches etc. Helps promote feelings of calmness during a stressful time. One three times a day for up to ten days.

## AROMATHERAPY

*Basil, Clary Sage, Lavender, Neroli, Palmarosa:* These oils all support the nervous system and will help impart a feeling of greater well-being. Combine in a base oil and massage in on a regular basis or use in the bath. Basil, although effective, should not be used for more than six weeks in any six-month period.

## STRETCH MARKS

Marks in the skin that form on fleshy parts such as thighs, buttocks, breasts and abdomen. They are formed when the skin has to accommodate weight loss or gain. Frequently occurring during pregnancy. There is an hereditary factor involved.

### HOMŒOPATHY

*Calc Fluor 6X:* Gives elasticity to the skin. One morning and night for ten days. This may be taken during pregnancy.

### AROMATHERAPY

*Frankincense (Olibanum), Mandarin, Neroli:* Combined in a base containing Wheatgerm Oil (as it contains vitamin E), and massaged daily onto affected areas, or during pregnancy to areas most likely to be affected.


## STYES

An infected boil or pimple on the eyelid without involvement of the eyeball and without any change in the vision of the eye. Inflammation erupts on the lid as a tender, red swelling. After a few days the stye usually comes to a head and discharges pus. Although sometimes painful, these are rarely dangerous, and can heal by themselves. Recurring styes can be an indication of general debility, and toxicity, and unexpressed anger (emotion).

### HERBS

*Eyebright, Marigold:* Combine, infuse and apply locally, as frequently as possible, or use diluted tinctures.

*Burdock, Echinacea, Eyebright, Red Clover:* Combine, infuse and drink three times daily for ten days. This will help to fight the infection and soothe the eyes.

### HOMŒOPATHY

*Apis 6 or 30:* Painful styes with burning and stinging. Eyelid becomes red and swollen; worse from heat. One dose of 30 potency a day for two days or one 6 three times a day for five days.

*Hepar Sulph 6 or 30:* Stye hypersensitive to touch and cold air; splinter sensation in the eyelid, pain relieved by warm applications. Dosage as for *Apis.*

*Pulsatilla 6 or 30:* Unsightly inflammation, but not particularly painful. Discharge of bland yellow or green pus. Itching. Dosage as for *Apis.*

*Silica 6X:* Morning and night for ten days. Styes that never come to a head, or leave a hard lump in the eyelid.

*Staphisagria 30:* Styes come out in groups or are recurrent. Irritable. Eye feels dry. Twice a day for three days.

AROMATHERAPY

*Lavender:* Soak cotton wool in a few drops mixed with warm water and hold over infected area taking care that none of the oil gets into the eye.


# SUNBURN AND SUNSTROKE

Exposure to the sun causes dehydration of the skin. To prevent painful burning and blistering, keep the skin protected with sunscreening lotions and only expose yourself to the sun for short periods of time until accustomed to it. In the event of burning treat as for burns. There are a variety of well tried and effective skin treatments: bathing in cool *Chamomile* infusion; applying a mixture of *Calendula* tincture and *Olive* oil; *Lavender* essential oil applied undiluted; *Aloe Vera* gel applied directly; *St John's Wort* oil or ointment applied directly; *Urtica* tincture or ointment applied directly.

If the person becomes severely overheated, the cooling mechanism of the skin fails and it becomes hot and dry. The body temperature can rise dangerously. The person may feel dizzy, nauseated, weak, feverish and have a severe headache. Treat for shock, seek emergency care, and cool the person off as quickly as possible with cold water until temperature begins to drop. Avoid over-chill-ing and give a glass of cold water with half a teaspoon of salt to encourage perspiration, and equalise balance of body fluids.

## HERBS
*Chickweed, Nettle, Peppermint:* A cooling combination of herbs. Make an infusion to drink as a tea or cool the infusion and bathe on an over-hot area.

## HOMŒOPATHY
*Belladonna 30:* Burning, dry, flushed skin. Feels feverish. Dilated pupils, throbbing headache. Two or three doses four hours apart.

*Glonoin 30:* Bursting, pounding headache after exposure to sun. Two or three doses four hours apart.

*Nat Mur 6X:* Several doses to encourage body fluids to return to normal.

## AROMATHERAPY
*Bergamot, Lavender:* Cooling and soothing oils to apply in a massage base or to add a few drops to a cool bath.

# T

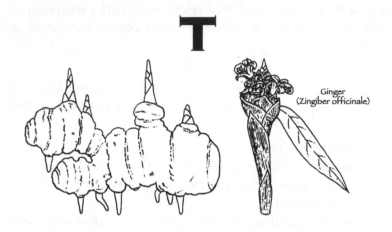

Ginger
(Zingiber officinale)

## TEETHING

Teething can be a distressing time for parents and infants. Teething symptoms vary according to the individual consitu-tion; common symptoms are flushed cheek, slightly raised temperature, peevishness, skin eruptions due to higher levels of acidity, gnashing of gums, and an increased tendency to earache. The following remedies may assist, but if symptoms persist constitutional treatment will be required. Teething symptoms may mask the beginning of another illness, so consult a practitioner if there is any doubt.

### HERBS

*Chamomile:* Make a weak infusion using one teaspoon of herb per half a pint of water. May be sweetened with honey if required. Allow the child to drink a tablespoon of infusion every four hours.

### HOMŒOPATHY

*Chamomilla 6 or 30:* Obtain in granule form or crush the tablet. Sprinkle a few granules or the powder onto the gums or into the mouth. Fretful, peevish child, one cheek flushed, sleepless, demands attention. Slight fever. Greenish stools. Take one dose every four hours while symptoms persist.

*Ferrum Phos 6X:* Crush the tablet and sprinkle the powder onto the gums. For redness and inflammation and slight feverishness. Take one dose every four hours while symptoms persist.

## THRUSH (CANDIDA)

Thrush is a yeast infection most commonly occurring in the mouth and the vagina, and can also occur in any folds of the skin, on the nipples, or in the bowel. Symptoms present with small red pimples becoming white patches, with a white discharge, itching and soreness in the area. This may be a sign of general debility, and sensitivity to fungal infections, or may be sexually transmitted. An increasingly common occurrence of thrush is after a course of antibiotics. Thrush in the mouth is most commonly found in babies, especially where there is an acid imbalance. It may be passed between the mouth and the nipple of the nursing mother. If vaginal thrush is aggravated by sexual contact, or if thrush is being passed between partners, then the use of a condom is advisable until the condition has improved.

The use of yogurt in the diet, and used externally, may be of benefit. Taking a probiotic supplement such as *Acidophilus* is also helpful. *Garlic* capsules or fresh *Garlic* have an anti-microbial effect on candida. If thrush is recurrent, constitutional treatment will be necessary, the following remedies may help relieve an acute episode.

### HERBS

*Golden Seal (half), Lavender, Marigold, Myrrh, Pau D'Arco, Thyme:* Combine and make an infusion for a vaginal douche. One dessertspoon of mixture to half a pint water. Leave standing until cool. Alternatively use the diluted tinctures. Soak a piece of cotton wool in the infusion and use to liberally bathe the area.

*Lavender, Myrrh:* Combine equal parts of the tinctures and dilute in warm water to use as a mouthwash for thrush in the mouth.

159

## HOMŒOPATHY

*Borax 30:* Thrush in the mouth. Patches of thrush and mouth ulcers that may bleed when touched. Infants mouth is hot and sore and causes difficulty feeding. One dose twice daily for five days.

*Kali Mur 6X:* White vaginal discharge or white coated tongue. Thrush in infants. Three times a day for ten days.

*Nat Phos, Nat Sulph, Silica 6X:* Symptoms of acidity. Use in combination with a douche to help eliminate thrush symptoms.

## AROMATHERAPY

*Lavender, Tea Tree:* Use externally. Add four drops of each to a sitz-bath.

# TONSILLITIS

Inflammation of the tonsils usually with streptoccocci bacteria present. It is most commonly found in children. Symptoms include: difficulty and pain when swallowing, white or red deposits on the tonsils and fever.

For an acute attack, treat as for fever and sore throat. Frequently recurring tonsillitis will require constitutional treatment from a qualified practitioner.

(See also: FEVER, SORE THROAT.)

# TOOTHACHE

We can only suggest a few first-aid measures to apply locally as it is necessary to be treated by your dentist who will treat the source of the pain.

*Calc Fluor 6X:* Improves enamel of teeth prone to rapid decay. This is particularly useful to take if you do not use a toothpaste containing fluoride and are prone to tooth decay. We recommend a course of *Calc Fluor*, one twice daily for ten days, two or three times a year.

## HERBS

*Marshmallow, Sage, Thyme:* Make a strong infusion (three teaspoons per cup) and use as a mouthwash to help soothe inflammation and counter infection.

*Cloves:* Chew a few of these to release the analgesic oil that they contain.

## HOMŒOPATHY

*Arnica 30:* Toothache following injury to the teeth or gums. Bruised soreness following a visit to the dentist. Two or three doses. Useful after tooth extraction.

*Belladonna 30:* Throbbing pain in the tooth or gum. Red, inflamed gum with signs of abscess. One dose three times a day.

*Ferrum Phos 6X:* Toothache with inflammation and soreness of gum, bleeding after extraction or after a blow to the area. One dose every two or three hours.

*Kali Phos 6X:* Severe pain in decayed or filled teeth, nagging dull toothache. One dose every two or three hours.

*Mag Phos 6X:* Severe toothache with shooting pains. Tooth sensitive to touch or cold air. One dose every two hours.

## AROMATHERAPY

*Clove:* Apply undiluted on cotton wool and place on affected area.

*Peppermint:* Though less effective, can be used in the same way.

These essential oils are not to be used for babies or young children.

## TRAVEL SICKNESS

A condition brought on by motion disturbing the balance mechanism within the inner ear, causing feelings of nausea and sometimes vomiting. There is also a psychological factor as nervous anticipation of travelling itself can cause similar reactions.

General advice is to have fresh air, frequent light digestible meals, and during travelling to lie or sit with the head slightly tilted backwards (as in a deck chair!).

### HERBS

*Ginger:* Chew the root, take ground *Ginger* in capsules, drink *Ginger* beer, or take diluted *Ginger* tincture before and during the journey.

*Meadowsweet, Peppermint Tinctures:* Combine and add ten drops to a cupful of water. Drink a cupful every few hours.

### HOMŒOPATHY

*Cocculus 30:* Severe nausea and vertigo. One dose before travel and repeat as necessary.

*Petroleum 30:* Dizziness and nausea aggravated by fumes. One dose before travel and repeat as necessary.

*Tabacum 30:* Boat sickness, worse if hot, severe nausea, violent vomiting. One dose before travel, and repeat as necessary.

### AROMATHERAPY

*Fennel, Ginger, Melissa, Peppermint:* Use the essential oil of your choice undiluted on cotton wool or a tissue and inhale frequently.

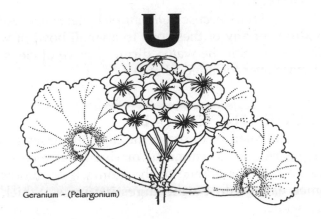

Geranium ~ (Pelargonium)

## ULCERS (EXTERNAL)

A persistent breach in a body surface. Their cause relies largely on where they are, but the failure to heal is the common link.

Varicose ulcers, found where there is poor circulation, are notoriously difficult to heal. Foot and leg exercises will help to encourage blood flow to the area. Professional medical care to advise about dressings is necessary. The following applications may also be tried for these and other slow-to-heal external lesions.

(See also: MOUTH ULCERS, VARICOSE VEINS.)

### HERBS

*Golden Seal (half), Echinacea, Hawthorn, Marigold, Shepherd's Purse, Yarrow:* Combine and make an infusion or use the tinctures to drink three times a day. This will stimulate circulation and promote healing.

*Comfrey Root, Marigold, Marshmallow:* A strong decoction or diluted tinctures of the above combination applied daily on clean lint to the area will reduce inflammation and promote healing.

### TINCTURES

*Calendula, Myrrh:* Dilute ten drops in a cupful of boiled water. Wash the affected part with cotton wool dipped in the solution. Repeat twice daily.

163

AROMATHERAPY

*Eucalyptus, Frankincense (Olibanum), Lavender:* Add a few drops of any of these oils to a small bowl of warm boiled water. Stir the water, dip in a piece of clean lint, and place over the affected area.

# ULCERS (INTERNAL)

Peptic ulcers refers to ulcers in the digestive tract, usually either gastric ulcers (stomach) or duodenal ulcers. Part of the mucous membrane of the stomach or duodenum becomes eaten into by the digestive juices which are highly acidic.

Emotional stress can promote a secretion of acid and is a cause of peptic ulcers. Other contributory factors are faulty diet (rich in fats and refined carbohydrates), smoking, stimulants, and alcohol.

The symptoms always include stomach pains, which may occur anywhere in the upper abdomen, but usually in the midline. The pain is generally ameliorated by vomiting and usually for a short time after eating. Heartburn and nausea are also common symptoms. Most peptic ulcers bleed at times and may cause anæmia. This condition may be extremely serious and complications include: sudden and severe bleeding, perforation of the stomach or duodenum and narrowing of the outlet of the stomach. Any persistent pain associated with the stomach should be referred to a medical practitioner for diagnosis as other diseases may show similar symptoms.

The following remedies will almost certainly bring relief to the painful symptoms, but unless one is prepared to change the lifestyle and particularly the level of stress and the diet, any remedies will only temporarily alleviate the symptoms without really getting to the cause of the problem. Professional advice may well be a necessary part of the healing process.

(See also: GASTRITIS.)

## HERBS

*Comfrey, Liquorice (half), Marigold, Marshmallow Root, Meadowsweet:* A combination of these herbs made into an infusion using a heaped teaspoon to a cupful of boiling water will promote healing, reduce acidity and relieve pain. Take three times a day for six weeks.

*Slippery Elm:* This is a highly nutritious food as well as providing a mucilaginous lining for the digestive tract. Regular use of this herb taken as a teaspoon stirred into a cupful of warm water will relieve pain and discomfort.

For nervine mixtures see ANXIETY.

## HOMŒOPATHY

Constitutional treatment by an experienced practitioner can be of definite aid in the healing of peptic ulcers.

## AROMATHERAPY

*Chamomile, Frankincense (Olibanum), Geranium, Marjoram:* Choose one or more of the above oils and add a few drops to a vegetable oil base. Massage into the abdomen. May be used in conjunction with other medication. Ideally, visit an aromatherapist for a relaxing and therapeutic massage.

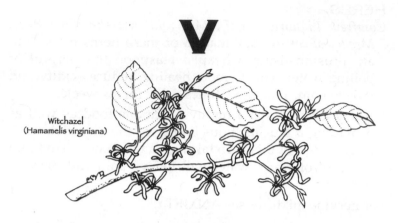

Witchazel
(Hamamelis virginiana)

## VAGINAL INFECTIONS

The symptoms of a vaginal infection are irritation and/or
an abnormal discharge. It is important to establish what
exacdy is causing the symptoms before treatment is possible, so seek medical advice. If a simple infection is diag-
nosed, treat as for THRUSH.

Vaginal infections are more common amongst women on
the pill or after menopause, because the secretions of hormones at this time do not offer the same protection.

(See also: MENOPAUSE, THRUSH.)

## VARICOSE VEINS

Swollen and distended veins in the leg caused by a combination of poor venous circulation, extra abdominal
pressure, e.g. constipation, water retention, obesity, pregnancy and a hereditary tendency. Prolonged periods of
standing and lack of exercise and smoking are contributory factors. General measures to improve the problem
include increased exercise, and a diet which will reduce
the tendency to constipation — a wholefood diet including plenty of fresh fruit and vegetables is recommended.
Resting with legs raised will help, together with giving
up smoking and drinking less tea.

Rutin will help to build up the walls of the veins; these can be taken as a bioflavonoid supplement or as buckwheat which is a main source of Rutin.

(See also: HAEMORRHOIDS.)

## HERBS

### EXTERNAL

*Marigold, Witchazel:* Can be made into a compress and used daily, or as a lotion applied onto the affected area.

### INTERNAL

*Horse Chestnut:* This is a specific for varicose veins – it is venotonic and aids venocongestion. It can be included in an internal mix (see below) as a tincture or applied externally as a lotion when combined with *Witchazel.*

*Dandelion Leaf, Hawthorn, Lime Blossom:* These herbs aid circulation, inflammation and are diuretic. Combine and make an infusion using one teaspoon per cup, or use as tinctures diluted in water. Drink three cups a day for up to four weeks. If no improvement is seen, consult a practitioner.

## HOMŒOPATHY

*Calc Fluor 6X:* To improve elasticity to the vein walls. Take one morning and night for ten days.

*Hamamelis 6:* Swollen, inflamed, painful, varicose veins, sore or prickling sensation in veins. Three times a day for a week.

## AROMATHERAPY

*Chamomile, Cypress, Lemon:* Combine, add a few drops to a light vegetable base oil and massage into legs around, rather than on, the veins, or use as a compress or in the bath.

## VOMITING

A reflex action with reversal of the normal movements of the muscles in the wall of the stomach. The reflex is clearly protective when it is set off by an irritant in the stomach or by overloading.

Repeated, forcible or sustained vomiting is always a serious symptom. It may indicate an emergency such as obstruction of the abdomen or poisoning, and it may lead to dehydration. Call emergency medical aid, whilst making sure the person is lying on their side so they cannot inhale the vomit, if they are unable to remain upright. Speed of action is essential with infants as they dehydrate so quickly.

For mild vomiting with an obvious cause, we suggest the following.

(See also: HANGOVERS, MORNING SICKNESS, NAUSEA, TRAVEL SICKNESS.)

### HERBS

*Balm, Chamomile, Meadowsweet:* Make an infusion of the above and sip the tea to reduce nausea and soothe the stomach.

### HOMŒOPATHY

*Aethusa 6 or 30:* Infant vomits their usual milk. Milk comes up in curds. If severe get immediate medical advice. Two or three doses.

*Ars Alb 6 or 30:* Vomiting and purging. Sips hot or cold drinks. Fearful and restless. Two or three doses.

*Bryonia 6 or 30:* Vomiting of solid food immediately after eating. Nausea and vomiting much better when lying absolutely still. Thirsty. Two or three doses as required.

*Ipecac 6 or 30:* Vomiting with constant nausea, not relieved by the vomiting. Clean tongue. Two or three doses as required.

*Nux Vomica 6 or 30:* Patient feels better for a while immediately after vomiting, then nausea builds up again;

worse after overloading the stomach; chilly and irritable. Two or three doses as required.

*Phosphorus 6 or 30:* Thirst for cold water that is vomited as soon as it reaches the stomach. Restless and anxious. Better for resting, burning in stomach. Two or three doses.

*Pulsatilla 6 or 30:* Stomach feels heavy. Aggravated by rich, fatty food. Thirstless. Feels sorry for themselves. Two or three doses.

## AROMATHERAPY

*Lavender, Peppermint, Roman Chamomile:* Add one or two drops of the oils to a vegetable base and massage into the abdomen or burn in the room.

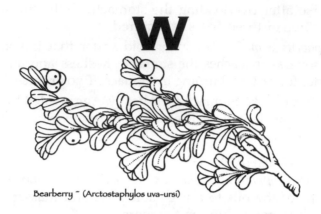

Bearberry ~ (Arctostaphylos uva-ursi)

# WARTS AND VERRUCAE

A wart is a growth on the skin that may be either hard or soft and fleshy. Warts are found in association with a virus which enters the body through a break in the skin, however, only a susceptible person will actually grow a wart which presents the probable need for constitutional treatment to properly eliminate the tendency to grow warts.

The most common sites for warts are fingers, knees, face and genitals.

Plantar warts (verrucae) are found on the soles of the feet and may become painful. They usually have a visible dark core. Treatment will be necessary to prevent them spreading.

The following remedies have been found to be successful where the warts are of a superficial nature. If they do not disappear, then the need for constitutional treatment to treat the tendency to produce warts is apparent.

HERBS

*Dandelion:* Squeeze the milky white sap from a stalk of fresh Dandelion onto the wart every day.

*Garlic:* Rub the wart with a slice from a peeled clove of Garlic every evening.

TINCTURES
*Thuja:* Dab on three times a day.

AROMATHERAPY
*Lemon, Tea Tree:* Dab on either of these oils, neat, twice daily.


# WATER RETENTION

Water retention is caused by the accumulation of fluid in the tissues. There are several distinct causes of water retention. In heart failure the water will accumulate in the legs, and in the cavity of the abdomen (ascites). Liver disease will cause water retention in the cavity of the abdomen. Salt retention will cause the tissues to retain more water; this is the cause of water retention associated with pregnancy or pre-menstrual tension where the change in hormone levels causes the body to retain more salt. Starvation and kidney disease will also cause water retention.

It becomes obvious that water retention is only curable by treating the cause and it is important to establish what the cause is. Salt will aggravate any water retention, therefore, a salt-free diet is advisable. The following remedies are comprised of some well-tried diuretics that may be used in consultation with your practitioner.

(See also: CELLULITE, CIRCULATION, JET LAG.)

HERBS
*Cornsilk, Dandelion, Uva Ursi, Yarrow:* Combine two or three of the above and make an infusion using a teaspoon of the herbs to a cup of boiling water. Drink three times daily. The most useful is probably *Dandelion* because it is naturally rich in potassium, and all diuretics tend to cause a loss of potassium from the body.

HOMŒOPATHY
Constitutional treatment must be sought.

## AROMATHERAPY
*Cypress, Juniper:* Dilute a few drops of each in a base oil to massage in, or add to the bath.

# WHOOPING COUGH
This is an infectious disease which affects the mucous membranes of the air passages, and usually occurs in children. The incubation period is around one week, and the initial symptoms are a sore throat and a cold.

After a week a violent, convulsive cough, which may be accompanied by vomiting, will occur. This can be very distressing, as during a coughing bout the child may not have time to draw in air and the 'whoop', so characteristic of the disease, is heard as the child struggles to inhale. This may not happen during a mild attack, but careful treatment and professional help should always be sought for whooping cough as damage can occur to the lungs or pneumonia may set in, especially in babies.

The following remedies must be used as an adjunct to medical supervision, and not replace it.

## HERBS
*Aniseed, Coltsfoot, Elecampane, White Horehound, Liquorice, Thyme:* Combine the above and make an infusion using two teaspoons of herbs to a cup of boiling water. Leave to stand for ten minutes, then strain and add honey to taste. Alternatively use the tinctures. Take three times a day.

Dosage

Babies: One teaspoon of infusion every four hours.

6 months to 5 years: Two teaspoons every four hours

Children over 5 years: One tablespoon every four hours.

## HOMŒOPATHY
*Bryonia 6 or 30:* Cough after eating and drinking. Child vomits. Dry, hard, painful cough, dreads the pain of the cough. One dose of 30th potency a day for three days, or three doses of 6th potency a day for five days.

*Carbo Veg 6 or 30:* Attacks of tormenting, choking cough. Face is flushed. Expectoration thick, yellow and profuse. Child craves fresh air. One dose of 30th potency a day for three days, or three doses of 6th potency a day for five days.

*Coccus Cacti 6 or 30:* Regular paroxysms of violent, tickling, racking cough ending in vomiting or raising of much clear, ropy mucus. Mucus hangs from the mouth. Purple face. Worse lying down. One dose of 30th potency a day for three days, or three doses of 6th potency a day for five days.

*Drosera 6 or 30:* Spasmodic, prolonged and incessant cough, followed by retching and vomiting. One dose of 30th potency a day for three days, or three doses of 6th potency a day for five days.

*Ipecac 6 or 30:* Cough violent and incessant. With every breath the child stiffens out, becomes blue or red in the face, and finally vomits. One dose of 30th potency a day for three days, or three doses of 6th potency a day for five days.

*Pertussin 30:* This is considered to be a homœopathic prophylactic against whooping cough. Give the child one dose a week during a whooping cough outbreak, or consult your practitioner. Also give this if other indicated remedies do not seem to be working well. One dose a day for three days.

Finding the right homœopathic remedy for whooping cough is not easy, and seeking professional guidance will bring the best results.

## AROMATHERAPY

*Cypress, Helichrysum, Ravensara, Thyme:* Place a few drops of one of the oils on a piece of cotton wool and put on the pillow near the child, or burn on an essential oil burner in the room. Alternatively, one or two of the oils may be added to a little base oil and rubbed onto the chest.

# WIND
(See: COLIC, FLATULENCE.)

# WORMS
The following treatment is recommended for thread-worms and roundworms, tapeworms must be treated professionally. Parasitic worms are a fairly common complaint, mostly in children. It is estimated that about 30 per cent of English children suffer from intestinal worms, mostly threadworms. These are passed on through oral infection from the anus where the worms lay their eggs. The life cycle of the egg in threadworms is about ten days, and so treatment must be aimed at breaking this cycle as well as alleviating the symptoms.

The symptoms of intestinal worms are irritability, boring of the nose with the fingers, and most markedly an itchy anus, which will be worse in the evening when the worms come out to lay their eggs. Diagnosis may be confirmed by observing the worms in the stools or around the anus in the evening.

Treatment requires scrupulous hygiene, paying particular attention to underwear, sheets and bed linen. The child should wear closely fitting underwear at night so they cannot inadvertently scratch the anus; wash the hands with hot soapy water, and scrub the nails after every visit to the lavatory. It will also be helpful to eat foods that the worms do not like, such as raw carrots, apples, onions, garlic and pumpkin seeds. Worms live on sugars so all foods containing sugar or even natural sweeteners such as malt or honey should be avoided.

*Calendula* ointment or Vaseline should be applied to the anus every evening to prevent the worms from laying their eggs and to relieve the itching.

## HERBS

Herbs which will kill worms are anthelmintics, these should be combined with a mild laxative to eliminate the worms.

*Liquorice (half), Quassia, Southernwood, Wormwood:* A very bitter but effective tea. Make a decoction and drink three times a day for three weeks. An enema of the herbs can be successful, but this is only advisable for adults.

## HOMŒOPATHY

*Cina 200:* Threadworms and roundworms. Twisting pains at the navel, itching at the anus, worse in the evenings. Irritable child, teeth grinding. One dose at bedtime, one the following morning; this may be repeated in ten days.

*Nat Phos 6X:* A course of this, one dose morning and night for ten days is a useful follow-up to either of the above remedies. It will help to rebalance the acid condition in the intestine, which becomes unbalanced with worms.

*Tellurium 30:* Itching is worse after passing stool. Pinching pains in abdomen. One dose a day for three days.

## AROMATHERAPY

*Eucalyptus, Lavender:* Add a couple of drops to vaseline and apply around the anus. This will prevent the worms from laying eggs.

# WRINKLES

Age, insomnia, weight loss, excessive sun, smoking, a hard life and hereditary tendencies (skin type), will all be significant in the development of wrinkles (or character lines).

It is the general level of mental and physical health which is most important to deal with. In order to lessen the process of forming wrinkles the following applications will help to allay the effects of ageing, and keep the skin supple:

*Rosehip Seed Oil:* A base oil with remarkable antioxidant properties. Repairs sun damage. Apply to the skin daily.

*Wheatgerm Oil:* This is rich in natural vitamin E which will help to keep the skin in good condition. Take two to four capsules a day, or apply the oil externally to the skin.

(See also: AGEING.)

AROMATHERAPY

*Cedarwood, Frankincense (Olibanum), Myrrh, Neroli, Patchouli:* Add a few drops of two or three of these oils to a light vegetable oil base and gently massage into the skin. A little *Wheatgerm* oil, *Rosehip Seed* oil or *Hazelnut* oil may also be added.

# APPENDIX
BACH FLOWER REMEDIES

The list below is intended as an aid to memory and for general enlightenment: it will not be sufficient information to prescribe from alone, otherwise disappointing results can ensue. See the Further Reading list for essential books on the subject, especially, "The Twelve Healers", which offers Dr Bach's original descriptions.

*Agrimony:* Worry hidden by a carefree mask, apparently jovial but suffering.

*Aspen:* Vague, unknown, haunting apprehensions and premonitions.

*Beech:* Intolerant, critical, fussy.

*Centaury:* Kind, quiet, gentle, anxious to serve, weak, dominated.

*Cerato:* Distrust of self and intuition, easily led and misguided.

*Cherry Plum:* For the thought of losing control, of doing dreaded things.

*Chestnut Bud:* Failing to learn from life, repeating mistakes, lack of observation.

*Chicory:* Self-pity, self-love, possessive, demanding, hurt and tearful.

*Clematis:* Dreamers, drowsy, absent-minded.

*Crab Apple:* Feeling unclean, self-disgust, small things out of proportion.

*Elm:* Capable people, with responsibility, who falter, temporarily overwhelmed.

*Gentian:* Discouragement, doubt, despondency.

*Gorse:* No hope, accepting the difficulty, pointless to try.

*Heather:* Longing for company, talkative, over-concern for self.

*Holly:* Jealousy, envy, revenge, anger, suspicion.

*Honeysuckle:* Living in memories.

*Hornbeam:* Feels weary and thinks can't cope.

*Impatiens:* Irritated by constraints, quick, tense, impatient.

*Larch:* Expect failure, lack confidence and will to succeed.

*Mimulus:* Fright of specific, known things: animals, heights, pain, etc., nervous, shy people.

*Mustard:* Gloom suddenly clouds us, for no apparent reason.

*Oak:* Persevering, despite difficulties, strong, patient, never giving in.

*Olive:* Exhausted, no more strength, need physical and mental renewal.

*Pine:* Self-critical, self-reproach, assuming blame, apologetic.

*Red Chestnut:* Worry for others, anticipating misfortune, projecting worry.

*Rock Rose:* Feeling alarmed, intensely scared, horror, dread.

*Rock Water:* Self-denial, stricture, rigidity, purist.

*Scleranthus:* Cannot resolve two choices, indecision, alternating.

*Star of Bethlehem:* For consolation and comfort in grief, after a fright or sudden alarm.

*Sweet Chestnut:* Unendurable desolation.

*Vervain:* Insistent, wilful, fervent, enthusiastic, stressed.

*Vine:* Dominating, tyrant, bully, demands obedience.

*Walnut:* Protection from outside influences, for change and the stages of development.

*Water Violet:* Withdrawn, aloof, proud, self-reliant, quiet grief.

*White Chestnut:* Unresolved, circling thoughts.

*Wild Oat:* Lack of direction, unfulfilled, drifting.

*Wild Rose:* Lack of interest, resignation, no love or point in life.

*Willow:* Dissatisfied, bitter, resentful, life is unfair, unjust.

*Five Flower Remedy:* Dr Bach chose five of the flower remedies as a combination, naming it 'rescue remedy'. This may be used in any kind of emergency, or in circumstances when we need immediate help, before and after moments of difficulty, and any kind of upset.

---

Printed with kind permission of Healing Herbs Ltd.

# SUPPLIERS

When purchasing items for medicinal purposes it is essential to use products of good quality.

Herbs, where possible, should be organically grown, and as fresh as possible.

Homœopathic remedies must be carefully prepared and stored.

Essential oils must be pure and of natural origin. Synthetic oils will not produce satisfactory therapeutic results, and may be damaging. Check with your retailer that their oils are definitely unadulterated essential oils.

All the products mentioned in this book are available from branches of Neal's Yard Remedies.

A mail order service is also available: 0845 262 3145 www.nealsyardremedies.com

In the USA most products should be available in good health food stores.

# CONTACTS

## HERBS:

To find a qualified herbalist in your area contact:
National Institute of Medical Herbalists,
56 Longbrook Street,
Exeter,
Devon EX4 6AH
Tel: (01392) 426022
www.nimh.org.uk

## HOMŒOPATHY:

To find a homoeopath in your area contact:

The Society of Homeopaths,
11 Brookfield, Duncan Close
Moulton Park,
Northampton NN3 6WL
Tel: 0845 450 6611

The Alliance of Registered Homeopaths,
Millbrook, Millbrook Hill,
Nutley,
East Sussex TN22 3PJ
Tel: 08700 736339
www.a-r-h.org

## AROMATHERAPY UK:

To find an aromatherapist in your area contact:
The Aromatherapy Consortium,
PO Box 6522,
Desborough, Kettering,
Northants NN14 2YX
Tel: 0870 774 3477

## BACH FLOWER REMEDIES
Healing Herbs of Dr Bach,
PO Box 65,
Hereford HR2 0DX
Tel: (01873) 890218
www.healingherbs.co.uk

## NUTRITION
British Association for Nutritional Therapy (BANT),
27 Old Gloucester Street,
London WC1N 3XX
Tel: 0870 606 1284
www.bant.org.uk

# FURTHER READING

HERBS

Barker, J., The Medicinal Flora, Kent: Winter Press, 2001.

Bartram, T., Encyclopedia of Herbal Medicine, England: Robinson, 1998.

Chevallier, A., The Encyclopedia of Medicinal Plants, London: Dorling Kindersley, 2001

Grieve, M., A Modern Herbal, London: Penguin, 1931.

Hoffman, D., The Holistic Herbal, Shaftesbury, Dorset: Element, 1983.


HOMŒOPATHY

Clarke, J.H., The Precriber, Saffron Walden, England: Health Science Press, 1972.

Cummings, S., Ullman, D., Everybody's Guide to Homeopathic Medicines, Los Angeles, USA: Tarcher, 1984.

Curtis, S., Homeopathic Alternatives to Immunisation, London: Winter Press, 1994.

Griffith, C., The Companion to Homoeopathy, London: Watkins, 2005.

Lessel, C.B., The Biochemic Handbook, Wellingborough, England: Thorsons, 1984.

Phatak, S.R., Materia Medica of Homœopathic Medicines, Delhi, India: IBPS, 1977.

Shepherd, D., Homœopathy for the First Aider, Saffron Walden, England: Health Science Press, 1945.

Speight, P., Before Calling the Doctor, Saffron Walden, England: Health Science Press, 1976.

Wells, R., Homoeopathy, London: Aurum, 2000.

AROMATHERAPY

Battaglia, S., The Complete Guide to Aromatherapy, Brisbane: ICHA, 2003.

Curtis, S., Essential Oils, London: Haldane Mason, 1996.

Davis, P., Aromatherapy: An A-Z, Saffron Walden, England: C.W. Daniel, 1988.

Tisserand, R., The Art of Aromatherapy, Saffron Walden, England: C.W. Daniel, 1977.


BACH FLOWER REMEDIES

Bach, E., Heal Thyself, Saffron Walden, England: C.W. Daniel, 1931.

Bach, E., Twelve Healers, Saffron Walden, England: C.W. Daniel, 1933.

Barnard, J., A Guide to the Bach Flower Remedies, Saffron Walden, England: C.W. Daniel, 1979.

Chancellor, P.M., Handbook of the Bach Flower Remedies, Saffron Walden, England: C.W. Daniel, 1971.

Wheeler, F.J., The Bach Remedies Repertory, Saffron Walden, England: C.W. Daniel, 1952.

# INDEX